KU-311-066

CONTENTS

OVERCOMING
ARTHRITIS

THE COMPLETE COMPLEMENTARY HEALTH PROGRAM

DR SARAH BREWER

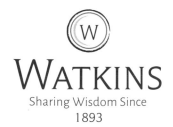

WATKINS
Sharing Wisdom Since
1893

Natural Health: Overcoming Arthritis

For my wonderful husband, Richard

This edition first published in the United Kingdom and Ireland in 2016 by
Watkins, an imprint of Watkins Media Limited
19 Cecil Court
London WC2N 4EZ

enquiries@watkinspublishing.com

Managing Editor: Grace Cheetham
Editors: Kesta Desmond, Sarah Epton, James Hodgson
Managing Designer: Suzanne Tuhrim
Commissioned artwork: Mark Watkinson

A CIP record for this book is available from the British Library

ISBN: 978-1-78028-103-2

10 9 8 7 6 5 4 3

Typeset in Ehrhardt and Calluna
Printed in Slovenia

Publisher's note:
The information in this book is not intended as a substitute for professional medical advice and
treatment. If you are pregnant or are suffering from any medical conditions or health problems,
it is recommended that you consult a medical professional before following any of the advice or
practices suggested in this book. Watkins Media Limited, or any other persons who have been
involved in working on this publication, cannot accept responsibility for any injuries or damage
incurred as a result of following the information, exercises, therapeutic techniques or recipes
contained in this book. The availability of some over-the-counter herbal remedies may be affected
by the 2004 EU Directive on Traditional Herbal Medicines. Consult a pharmacist or qualified
herbal practitioner for advice on this subject.

Notes on the recipes
Unless otherwise stated: use medium eggs, fruit and vegetables. Use fresh ingredients, including
herbs. Do not mix metric and imperial measurements.
1tsp = 5ml, 1tbsp = 15ml, 1 cup = 250ml

www.watkinspublishing.com

INTRODUCTION

Arthritis is the inflammation of one or more joints and it comes in a variety of forms. All cause similar symptoms of pain, swelling, stiffness and restriction of movement, which can have a major effect on quality of life. Worldwide, as many as one in two people over the age of 60 have self-reported arthritis symptoms. These symptoms may be mild and intermittent or they may be severe and continuous. The number of people in the UK affected by arthritis is around seven million. In the US, an estimated 40 million people have arthritis, and the number is expected to reach 59 million by the year 2020. In Australia, more than three-and-a-half million people have arthritis, and this figure is expected to increase to seven million by 2050.

Although it becomes more common with advancing age, joint problems affect younger people, too. Around 25 people in a thousand aged under 40 have arthritis, with juvenile arthritis affecting between one and four out of every thousand children in different countries.

The good news is that many cases of arthritis can be relieved, postponed or even prevented by good joint care – that's my aim in writing this book. Many of us tend to take our joints for granted until they start playing up, by which time significant damage may already have occurred. The sooner you start looking after your joints, the better. If any of the following apply to you, I recommend that you start to make diet and lifestyle changes now:

FOLLOW YOUR DOCTOR'S ADVICE

The information and advice given in this book is for general information only. It's not intended to replace individual advice from your own doctor. My approach is holistic and designed to complement the treatments your doctor prescribes. If you follow one or more of the programs in Part Three, please treat my advice as a guide only and always follow the advice of your doctor or other healthcare professionals who know your specific needs in detail. In particular, never stop taking your arthritis medication except under the advice and supervision of your own doctor.

- You are aged 40 or over.
- Arthritis runs in your family.
- You are overweight.
- You take little regular exercise.
- Your work involves repetitive movements of one or more joints.
- You feel the need to stretch your back every day.
- You notice creakiness in one or more joints.
- You notice that a joint, such as your knee or hip, is less flexible than before, or cannot be straightened fully.
- You can no longer touch your toes when standing with knees straight.
- You have limited neck rotation and can no longer align your chin with your shoulder tip, or touch the front of your chest with your chin.
- Your joints are swelling or changing shape.
- Your fingers and toes easily get cold and stiff.
- A joint starts aching, especially after exercise.
- Your knees are painful when you kneel or sit on them.

Many people with joint pain avoid exercise but, as discussed on pages 97–103, regular exercise is vitally important for long-term joint health. If you have arthritis, your joints will need *some* rest, but too much will make your muscles weak and increase your joint stiffness. Simple exercises, such as stretching, walking, cycling or swimming, can go a long way to keep your joints healthy and flexible. If you're overweight, your weight-bearing joints will have to work harder than they would otherwise – I explain how you can lose weight on pages 103–105.

Like your heart, your joints thrive best on a healthy lifestyle and a diet that is rich in superfoods (see pages 82–86). In Part Three I show you how you can change your lifestyle and diet for maximum benefit. Because everyone is different and no diet and lifestyle plan will suit all individuals, I've created three different approaches: a gentle, a moderate and a full-strength program. To help you work out which one is right for you, complete the questionnaire on pages 109–110.

For many people, the gentle program is a good place to start. It introduces you to healthy eating principles such as eating more fruit, vegetables and fish. I suggest you take food supplements such as glucosamine at a dose that will have a significant, beneficial effect on your arthritis symptoms. I also show you some useful stretch exercises, and introduce you to complementary health approaches such as aromatherapy and homeopathy. A month on the gentle program can significantly reduce the level of inflammation in your joints.

If your responses to the questionnaire suggest that you have a sensitivity to plants of the nightshade family, such as tomatoes, peppers, chillies, aubergines, and potatoes, the moderate program shows you how to exclude these foods from your diet. I also provide some stretch and range-of-movement exercises, and introduce you to complementary approaches such as reflexology and meditation. If you're sensitive to foods from the nightshade family, you should notice your symptoms becoming less troublesome within a month of following the moderate program.

For people whose questionnaire identifies a pronounced inflammatory component to their arthritis, the full-strength program will provide an eating plan that significantly increases your intake of antioxidants and spices with a natural, analgesic action. I also include an exercise program to help you to stay active and flexible; and I introduce you to complementary techniques such as acupressure and acupuncture. If your arthritis is linked with inflammatory reactions within your joints, the full-strength program has the potential to relieve symptoms within a month.

LOOK OUT FOR THESE SYMBOLS

Throughout this book I have included boxes that highlight useful, interesting or important pieces of information. Each box bears a symbol (see below). The arrow symbol indicates that a box contains practical instructions. The plus sign means that the box contains additional information about the subject being discussed or about asthma in general. The exclamation mark indicates a warning or a caution.

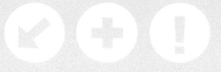

PART ONE
UNDERSTANDING ARTHRITIS

A condition that appears in many guises, arthritis can take the form of osteoarthritis, which is linked to increasing age, and wear and tear on the joints; or it can be a condition such as rheumatoid arthritis and psoriatic arthropathy in which the body's own immune system attacks the joints. Gout is another type of arthritis. Whichever type you have, the underlying symptoms are essentially the same – joint pain, stiffness, swelling and restricted movement. To help you understand the nature of arthritis I describe the different types of joint in the human body and the different types of arthritis that can affect them. Although the causes of arthritis are not yet fully understood, I explain the current understanding of the genetics that underlie autoimmune arthritis, and the factors that can damage joints and lead to osteoarthritis. Your doctor will diagnose which type of arthritis you have using a range of techniques – for example, physical examination, x-rays and analysis of your joint fluid. A number of diagnostic blood tests are also available. I explain the variety of painkilling and immune-modifying drugs that can help to control your symptoms. I also describe the variety of different approaches that orthopedic surgery can offer.

WHAT IS ARTHRITIS?

The word arthritis means inflammation of a joint. A joint forms where two bones come into close contact with each other. Some joints have limited flexibility and are designed to allow for growth, such as those in the skull which fuse together to form suture joints only after the skull is fully mature. Other joints have a limited amount of movement to absorb shock, and are stabilized by pads of cartilage, such as those between the two long bones in your lower leg (the tibia and fibula). However, most joints can move more freely through a variable range of movements. To fully understand what happens when arthritis develops, it's useful to have an understanding of the joints and their surrounding structures.

UNDERSTANDING YOUR JOINTS

There are six different types of moveable joint, all of which can be affected by arthritis.

In a ball-and-socket joint, a round-shaped bone surface fits inside a cup-shaped socket in another bone. This type of joint, such as the hip, has the greatest range of movement. The shoulder ball-and-socket joint has the widest range of movement of all. It's known as a multiaxial joint, as the arm can move in more than two planes: up and down, backward and forward plus rotating in a circle at the side of the body.

Ellipsoid joints consist of an oval-shaped bone surface fitting into an oval-shaped cup in another bone. This type of joint, such as the wrist, can move back and forth or from side to side, but full rotation is limited.

In a saddle joint, two U-shaped bone surfaces fit together at right angles to rock back and forth and from side to side. This joint gives the thumb limited rotation.

Hinge joints consist of the cylindrical surface of one bone sitting inside the curve of another. A hinge joint, such as that of the fingers, allows movement in one plane. The elbow and knee are examples of modified hinge joints.

In a pivot joint, one bone swivels inside a space formed by another bone. The pivot joint between two upper neck vertebrae (the axis and atlas) allows the head to swivel from side to side.

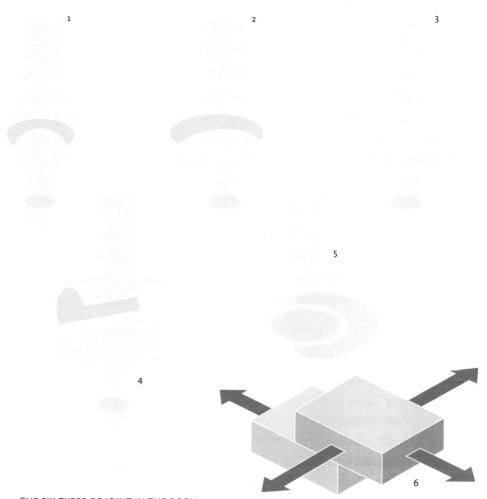

THE SIX TYPES OF JOINT IN THE BODY
1. Ball and socket (hip); 2. Ellipsoid (wrist);
3. Saddle (thumb); 4. Hinge (elbow); 5. Pivot (upper neck);
6. Gliding (some joints in the spine, hands and feet)

Finally, in a gliding joint, two joint surfaces that are almost flat move by sliding over each other. Some of the joints in the vertebral column, hands and feet are of this kind, and are bound together by strong ligaments that limit their range of movement.

Your joints are made of other elements too:

LIGAMENTS

Joints are bound together by tough, slightly elastic bands of collagen fibre known as ligaments. These form a capsule around a mobile joint and provide reinforcement. Some joints, such as the knee, also have internal ligaments for additional stability, allowing the joint to bend while stopping the ends of the bones from moving back and forth, or side to side. People described as "double-jointed" have a wider range of joint movement than usual as a result of inheriting looser, more elastic ligaments (known as hyperlaxity).

CARTILAGE

This slippery substance protects the surfaces of mobile joints from wear and tear by allowing the bones to slide easily over one another. Discs of cartilage are found in the knee joints and where the jaw bone articulates (forms a joint) with the skull. These discs of articular cartilage act like washers to reduce friction between moving bones. Cartilage contains collagen and elastin fibres plus a tough, gel-like substance, called the matrix, which is secreted by embedded cells called chondrocytes.

SYNOVIAL FLUID

The capsule of a mobile joint is lined with a thin tissue called the synovial membrane. This secretes a thick, slippery fluid that resembles egg white. Synovial fluid cushions and oils the joints, provides them with nutrients and reduces friction between the articular cartilage.

TENDONS

Joints are moved by the relaxation and contraction of opposing groups of muscle, which attach to the bones via elastic strands of tissue known as tendons. The tendons run within oiled tubes, known as sheaths.

BURSAE

These are fluid-filled sacs above and below certain joints, such as the knee. They store synovial fluid, and act as cushions to prevent tendons and muscles from rubbing at pressure points.

TYPES OF ARTHRITIS

There are many different types of arthritis – the most common type is osteoarthritis followed by rheumatoid arthritis.

OSTEOARTHRITIS (OA)

This involves degeneration of the cartilage that protects the bone ends within a joint. Without cartilage protection, the bone ends rub together and become inflamed. As the cartilage becomes pitted, cracked and flaky, synovial fluid leaks through the cracks into the underlying bone. The causes the bone to thicken and become mildly inflamed, forming small cysts and bony swellings called osteophytes. The bone ends may eventually rub together. The synovial membrane and joint capsule also thicken and the space inside the joint becomes increasingly narrow. As a result of all these processes, joint movements become painful, stiff and restricted, and affected joints may change in appearance – they may start to look knobbly and enlarged. Walking awkwardly causes associated ligaments and muscles to ache, and joint pain often keeps you awake at night. You may feel or hear creaking and cracking as you move, and your muscles may become wasted from lack of use. Osteoarthritis usually affects larger, weight-bearing joints such as the hips, knees and lower spine, but it can also affect other mobile joints such as the neck, shoulders, elbows, wrists, ankles, fingers, toes and jaw.

RHEUMATOID ARTHRITIS

This develops when your immune system wrongly identifies parts of a joint as "foreign" and attacks them. The synovial membrane lining certain joints becomes inflamed owing to abnormal activity of certain immune cells (T and B lymphocytes). Inflammation gradually spreads from the synovial membrane to the tendon sheaths, and the membrane lining the bursae (see page 14–15) around affected joints. Eventually, the bone may be affected, too, to cause characteristic joint deformities such

JOINTS AFFECTED BY ARTHRITIS
Osteoarthritis begins with a deterioration in the cartilage in your joints. This is usually followed by damage to the bone and synovial membrane. Rheumatoid arthritis begins with the inflammation of the synovial membrane, followed by cartilage and bone destruction.

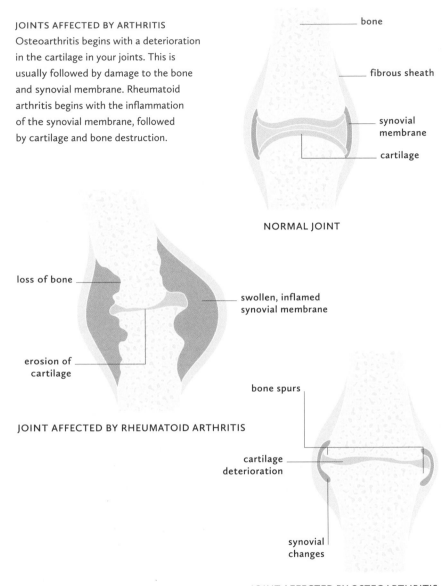

bone

fibrous sheath

synovial membrane

cartilage

NORMAL JOINT

loss of bone

swollen, inflamed synovial membrane

erosion of cartilage

JOINT AFFECTED BY RHEUMATOID ARTHRITIS

bone spurs

cartilage deterioration

synovial changes

JOINT AFFECTED BY OSTEOARTHRITIS

as those in the hands, in which the fingers deviate toward the little finger. Rheumatoid arthritis usually affects the smaller joints in the wrists, hands and feet, but can also occur in the neck, knees and ankles. It usually develops symmetrically so that the same joints on both sides of the body become red, hot and swollen. Early morning stiffness that lasts for several hours is common, as are weight loss, fever and exhaustion. Rheumatoid arthritis tends to be a remitting and relapsing disease in which flare-ups are followed by periods in which symptoms improve. The autoimmune process can also attack other parts of the body, including the skin, muscles, blood vessels, heart, lungs and eyes. Because of its widespread, systemic nature, people with rheumatoid arthritis are also more likely to experience a heart attack or stroke than others – probably because inflammation affects the circulation and thickens the blood, too. If you have rheumatoid arthritis, it's important to have regular cardiovascular checks. Children can also develop rheumatoid arthritis – when it affects people who are under the age of 16, it's known as juvenile rheumatoid arthritis or Still's disease.

OTHER TYPES OF ARTHRITIS

Joint inflammation may be the result of autoimmune disease, such as psoriasis, lupus and inflammatory bowel disease, as well as the following:

- Gout – a form of arthritis in which needle-like crystals of a substance called uric acid are deposited in a joint, typically at the base of the big toe. It can also manifest in other small joints in the feet and hands – especially the thumb – as well as in larger joints such as the knee, ankle or wrist. Uric acid crystals cause severe inflammation and exquisite tenderness with redness and swelling of the affected joint. Mild fever may also occur.
- Pseudogout – this is similar to gout, but calcium pyrophosphate, rather than uric acid, is deposited within a joint, most often the knee, although also the wrist, shoulder, ankle, elbow and hand.
- Septic arthritis – this is when a joint is infected by bacteria, a virus or even certain fungi. Most cases involve the skin bacteria *Staphylococcus aureus*.
- Reactive arthritis – this results from infections that do not directly involve the joint. It's also known as post-exposure arthritis, and it occurs when antibodies made to fight an infection in one part of the

body attack the joints as if they were also infected, when they are not. This form of immune attack most commonly affects people who carry a gene known as human lymphocyte antigen B27 (HLA-B27). Reactive arthritis can occur following gastroenteritis (food poisoning) with organisms such as salmonella, campylobacter, clostridium, shigella and *Entamoeba histolytica*. It can also follow genitourinary infections such as chlamydia or gonorrhea. Lyme disease is also more likely to cause reactive arthritis than septic arthritis.

- Ankylosing spondylitis – also more common in people carrying the HLA-B27 gene, this is a form of autoimmune disease in which inflammation affects the sacroiliac joints in the pelvis, and small joints within the vertebral column that may eventually fuse. It can also affect the hips, knees and shoulders. Other symptoms include loss of appetite, tiredness, feeling unwell, and inflammation of the iris in the eye (iritis).
- Psoriatic arthropathy – this is a form of autoimmune arthritis that affects between 10 and 20 percent of people with psoriasis (an inflammatory skin disease). There's no link between the severity of skin symptoms and whether or not your joints are affected. As with other forms of autoimmune arthritis, the synovial membrane becomes inflamed and releases more fluid than normal, and the joint becomes tender and swollen. As inflammation continues, it spreads to the cartilage underneath and may eventually erode the bone. As the tendons are lined and lubricated by a synovial membrane, these also become inflamed, especially around the elbows, wrists and heels. The most common type of psoriatic arthropathy involves the small joints of the fingers and toes, producing sausage-shaped digits. Pitting of the nails and inflammation of the sacroiliac joints in the pelvis are also common.

CAUSES, SIGNS AND SYMPTOMS

Although there are many different types of arthritis, with many different underlying causes, the basic symptoms and signs of joint damage are similar in every case.

WHY ARTHRITIS DEVELOPS

The reasons why some people develop arthritis while others don't is not fully understood, but is believed to result from interactions between a number of factors, including heredity, lifestyle and environment.

GENES

All types of arthritis appear to run in families and are likely to involve certain genes. For example, it makes sense that if you inherit a weaker or thinner layer of articular cartilage (see pages 14), you're likely to be more prone to osteoarthritis. And genetic mutation affecting collagen production has been linked with the premature breakdown of joint cartilage in some families. Researchers have also found that genes that affect communication between cartilage-making cells (chondrocytes) influence your susceptibility for developing osteoarthritis of the hip. Overall, it's thought that 60 percent of osteoarthritis has a genetic basis, and 25 percent of cases result from a single, specific, gene mutation.

One of the strongest hereditary links with arthritis involves the gene HLA-B27, which codes for a specific protein on the surfaces of white blood cells. If you inherit this gene, you're four times more likely than normal to develop reactive arthritis, psoriatic arthropathy or ankylosing spondylitis. But, although 90 percent of people with ankylosing spondylitis carry the HLA-B27 gene, only two to six percent of those with HLA-B27 develop ankylosing spondylitis. This suggests that another trigger is needed; for example, inheriting other associated genes, or exposure to an environmental trigger, such as a specific infection.

Researchers have found that inheriting another gene involved in cell "self" recognition, called HLA-DR4, significantly increases the risk of developing rheumatoid arthritis, psoriatic arthritis and reactive arthritis following Lyme disease.

Among identical twins, if one twin develops an autoimmune type of arthritis, such as rheumatoid arthritis, the chance that the other twin will develop it is only 15 to 30 percent, suggesting that non-genetic factors, such as exposure to a virus, are necessary for the disease to express itself. Twenty percent of people with gout have a family history of the disease.

INFECTION

A joint damaged by direct infection (septic arthritis) is likely to develop osteoarthritis in the future. Infection may also trigger autoimmune arthritis in some people. For example, people with rheumatoid arthritis appear to have higher levels of antibodies against the Epstein-Barr virus than people without.

GENDER

Women are five times more likely to develop rheumatoid arthritis than men, but men are three times more likely to develop ankylosing spondylitis than women, and to have it more severely. This suggests that some forms of arthritis have causes that are sex-linked (perhaps carried on the X or Y chromosomes that determine sex) or are in some way affected by male or female hormones (testosterone or oestrogen). For example, gout is nine times more common in men than women because oestrogen promotes the excretion of uric acid crystals into urine.

AGE

Osteoarthritis usually develops over many years, probably because the water content of cartilage decreases with age, and it becomes more brittle and less easy to repair. Most over-65s have osteoarthritis in at least one joint, although only 30 percent of those with x-ray evidence of osteoarthritis have pain at the relevant site. Autoimmune diseases also tend to start at specific times of life – for example, ankylosing spondylitis tends to develop between 16 and 30 years of age, and seldom in people over the age of 40. Similarly, a quarter of people with rheumatoid arthritis develop symptoms before the age of 30, and most new cases occur in the 40 to 50 age group. And in four out of five children with juvenile rheumatoid arthritis, symptoms disappear before the age of 20. Age is undoubtedly implicated in the cause of arthritis, but there need to be other triggers too.

EXCESS WEIGHT

Being overweight greatly increases the risk of osteoarthritis in weight-bearing joints. This is because joint damage is partly dependent on the load the joint has to support. As a result, someone who is overweight is seven times more likely to develop osteoarthritis of the knee than someone in the healthy weight range for their height.

PREVIOUS JOINT DAMAGE

People who put excessive strain on their joints in early life (for example, athletes), or those who have previously injured their joints through accidents or sport, are at increased risk of developing osteoarthritis in later life. A joint previously damaged by septic arthritis or recurrent episodes of gout is also likely to progress to osteoarthritis, as a result of irregularities on the surface of cartilage.

WHAT ARE THE SYMPTOMS?

The main signs and symptoms of arthritis are localized pain, tenderness, redness, hotness, swelling, stiffness and loss of movement. They may be acute or chronic (long term). Acute joint inflammation resolves once the immediate cause is removed, such as the infecting organisms in the case of septic arthritis, or the crystals deposited in gout or pseudogout. Chronic inflammation occurs in osteoarthritis, where articular cartilage remains thin and brittle, and in autoimmune arthritis, where immune

WHY DO JOINTS GET INFLAMED?

Inflammation is an important part of the body's healing process – it occurs when immune cells congregate to destroy tissues that are infected or diseased. When a patrolling white blood cell enters a joint and identifies something as wrong, it secretes a number of chemical alarm signals known as cytokines. These attract other immune cells into the area and super-stimulate them, so they are ready to fight infection or destroy damaged or abnormal body cells. Histamine is also released, which causes small blood vessels to dilate and become more permeable – bringing in blood and nutrients while flushing away toxins. The body also produces chemicals that stimulate pain receptors – nature's way of making you rest and immobilize a joint while healing occurs. All these reactions are responsible for the characteristic symptoms of an arthritis flare-up.

cells continue to misidentify the synovial membrane as foreign. Abnormal immune reactions also account for the tiredness and fatigue that typically accompany autoimmune diseases.

DIAGNOSING ARTHRITIS

Your doctor will look at your joints and listen to a description of your symptoms as part of the diagnosis of arthritis. He or she is also likely to use x-rays, blood tests and other investigative techniques to help to identify the cause of your joint pain.

CASE HISTORY

Your doctor will ask you about your symptoms and which joints are affected. Morning stiffness that goes within 30 minutes, or stiffness that comes on later in the day after repetitive use, is usually a result of osteoarthritis, but morning stiffness that lasts longer than 30 minutes is more typical of rheumatoid arthritis. If non-symmetrical joints are affected (for example, one hip, one knee, one hand), then osteoarthritis is the most likely diagnosis, but if your joint symptoms are symmetrical (for example, both hands or wrists, both knees), this suggests rheumatoid arthritis, especially if your joints are red, swollen, warm and tender.

HOW MANY JOINTS ARE AFFECTED?

The number of painful joints can be an indication of which type of arthritis you have. Pain that affects a single joint is known as monoarthritis. This is usually characteristic of osteoarthritis, trauma, infection (septic arthritis) or a crystalline arthritis (gout or pseudogout). Pain involving two, three or four joints is called oligoarthritis and suggests either osteoarthritis or an autoimmune condition such as rheumatoid arthritis or psoriatic arthropathy. Pain affecting five or more joints is referred to as polyarthritis. This is indicative of a widespread, autoimmune disorder, such as rheumatoid arthritis, psoriatic arthritis, or joint involvement in another autoimmune condition such as lupus (an ulcerative skin disease).

Your doctor will also ask about any previous personal history relating to your joints, such as injury, and about your family history of arthritic conditions.

PHYSICAL EXAMINATION

During an examination, a doctor will assess how red, swollen and warm your joints are and whether there is a build up of fluid (effusion) within the joint. He or she will also look for the following:

- Bony or soft tissue nodules. Heberden's nodes and Bouchard's nodes are bony nodules that frequently develop around the joints of the fingers in older people with osteoarthritis, while people with rheumatoid arthritis develop rheumatoid nodules under the skin, especially at the elbow and down the forearm.
- The characteristic deformities of rheumatoid arthritis, such as boutonnière and swan-neck deformities of the fingers (see page 25), owing to erosion of finger joints, tendons and ligaments. The fingers may also deviate toward the little finger owing to destruction of the knuckle joints.
- Unusually marked muscle wasting (this is characteristic of rheumatoid arthritis).
- Swellings, called tophi, caused by a build up of uric acid crystals. They may erode through the skin in white, chalky nodules. Tophi are a sign of gout.
- Pin-prick depressions in the fingernails – called pitting – which are a sign of psoriatic arthropathy.
- Limited movement in any of the joints.
- "Crunching" or an audible sound when you move a joint.

X-RAYS

If you have osteoarthritis, x-rays of the affected joint may show a characteristic narrowing and irregularity of the joint space, as well as bone changes, such as increased density in the bone ends, formation of bony lumps (osteophytes) and "holes" in the bone beneath the cartilage, known as pseudocysts. However, lack of these findings does not mean that you definitely do not have osteoarthritis. Similarly, some people may have x-ray findings consistent with osteoarthritis, but have no symptoms or disability.

LABORATORY TESTS

Laboratory tests on samples of blood or other body fluids can help differentiate between different types of arthritis, and can also help monitor disease activity and the effectiveness of treatment once a diagnosis is established.

FULL BLOOD COUNT

This gives a complete analysis of the white blood cells, red blood cells, platelets (clotting cell fragments) and the amount of red blood pigment (hemoglobin) present in your blood. A raised white-blood-cell level suggests that an active infection is present; low levels of white blood cells, red blood cells and hemoglobin suggest that you may have a chronic inflammatory disease, such as rheumatoid arthritis.

ERYTHROCYTE SEDIMENTATION RATE (ESR)

This measures how quickly your red blood cells clump together and fall down a glass column. ESR is measured in millimetres per hour. A level above 100mm/hr is an indication of abnormal inflammation that is usually autoimmune or infective in nature.

C-REACTIVE PROTEIN (CRP)

This is a "sticky" protein produced by the liver as part of the body's inflammatory response. Your CRP level is a more sensitive marker of inflammation than ESR, so doctors are increasingly using this test. Levels of 3mg/L or higher are considered raised.

ANTIBODY BLOOD TESTS

A raised level of antibodies suggests an infection or an autoimmune response.

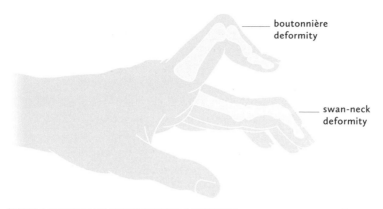

boutonnière
deformity

swan-neck
deformity

HAND AFFECTED BY RHEUMATOID ARTHRITIS

Herberden's node

Bouchard's node

HOW ARTHRITIS AFFECTS THE FINGER JOINTS
Sometimes the appearance of your joints is sufficient
to diagnose arthritis. For example, bony nodules at the
finger joints may be a sign of osteoarthritis; and finger
deformities may be a sign of rheumatoid arthritis.

HAND AFFECTED BY OSTEOARTHRITIS

ANTI-NUCLEAR ANTIBODIES (ANA)

These are abnormal autoantibodies aimed against parts of the nucleus
found in the centre of all cells of the body except for red blood cells.
Moderate to high antinuclear antibody levels suggest an autoimmune
disease, and are usually found in 30 to 50 percent of people with
rheumatoid arthritis.

WHAT IS ARTHROCENTESIS?

When a single joint is inflamed and swollen, a doctor may take a sample of the joint fluid using a sterile needle and syringe under local anesthetic. Normal joint fluid is slightly sticky (viscous) and is either crystal clear or a light straw colour. If the fluid is cloudy this is a sign of inflammation. If there is obvious pus in the fluid, this suggests septic arthritis. Laboratory analysis of joint fluid can detect the presence of protein, white blood cells, red blood cells, bacteria and crystals. If the joint fluid forms a clot within one hour of collection, this indicates the presence of a clotting protein fibrin, which is characteristic of inflammation of the synovial membrane.

RHEUMATOID FACTOR (RF)

This is an antibody found in around 80 percent of people with rheumatoid arthritis and about one percent of healthy people without rheumatoid arthritis. However, it's not fully diagnostic as RF is also found in some people with other autoimmune conditions, such as lupus; in people with long-term viral infections, such as chronic hepatitis; and in some people with leukemia.

ANTI-CYCLIC CITRULLINATED PEPTIDE (ANTI-CCP)

This is an antibody aimed against an unusual amino acid called citrulline. Chains of amino acids that include citrulline are found in joints affected by rheumatoid arthritis but not other forms of arthritis. Its presence means there is a 95 percent chance that you have rheumatoid arthritis.

HLA-TISSUE TYPING

Some types of autoimmune arthritis are more likely in people with certain genes such as HLA-B27 and HLA-DR4 (see page 19). If your joint symptoms are difficult to diagnose, it can help to know whether or not you carry these genes.

URIC ACID LEVEL

If gout is suspected, a high level of uric acid in the blood helps to confirm the diagnosis.

OTHER TESTS

You may need a range of other tests during the diagnosis of an inflamed joint, including computed axial tomography (CAT) or magnetic resonance imaging (MRI) scans. These produce detailed, cross-sectional images of the internal structures of a joint. Arthroscopy, in which a small optic tube (arthroscope) is inserted into the joint under general anesthetic, also allows direct viewing of the joint to evaluate degenerative changes and to determine the cause of pain and inflammation. A relatively new procedure, thermal imaging, can show the degree of inflammation by measuring changes in temperature across the joints.

TREATING ARTHRITIS

The medical treatment of all types of arthritis initially involves painkillers, such as paracetamol, and non-steroidal anti-inflammatory drugs (NSAIDs), such as ibuprofen. You may also be offered physiotherapy. In addition, some forms of arthritis require disease-modifying drugs that damp down abnormal immune reactions. If your joint symptoms aren't relieved by drug therapy and physiotherapy, you may need joint replacement surgery.

PAINKILLERS

Pain is a subjective, unpleasant sensation that's associated with actual or potential tissue damage. Because it's subjective, and can't be measured directly, your doctor relies heavily on your description of pain to select the right strength of drug. He or she may ask you to rate your pain on a scale of zero to 10: zero is no pain and 10 is the worst pain imaginable.

PARACETAMOL (ACETAMINOPHEN)

This is the most widely used analgesic for arthritis as it's effective for mild to moderate pain and has the least potential to cause adverse side effects when used at the correct dose of no more than 1g, every four to six hours, up to a maximum dose of 4g daily. Paracetamol has a direct effect on the brain to kill pain and lower fever, but it doesn't have an anti-inflammatory action and doesn't reduce stiffness. It's therefore most helpful for osteoarthritis in which joint inflammation is minimal. Check with a doctor before taking paracetamol if you have kidney or liver problems. Don't take more than one product containing paracetamol at a time.

ASPIRIN (ACETYLSALICYLIC ACID)

This is effective against mild to moderate pain and it reduces fever. It works by blocking the production of inflammatory chemicals in the body through the inhibition of an enzyme known as cyclo-oxygenase-1 (COX-1). It's suitable for most types of arthritis, especially those associated with inflammation, but it's usually avoided in cases of gout because it can increase the blood level of uric acid to precipitate an attack in some people. Aspirin is best taken in soluble, effervescent or enteric-coated form to minimize stomach irritation. It's not usually advised for children under the age of 16, for pregnant or breastfeeding women, or for people with a history of peptic ulcers, asthma or a blood-clotting disorder. Check with a doctor before taking aspirin if you have gout, asthma, kidney or liver problems, or if you are on any other medication (drug interactions are common).

BENORILATE

This is a chemical cross between paracetamol and aspirin: 2g benorilate contains just over 1g of aspirin, and just under 1g paracetamol. It's effective against mild to moderate pain.

NON-STEROIDAL ANTI-INFLAMMATORY DRUGS (NSAIDS)

In single or low doses, NSAIDs act as painkillers, and have a similar effect to paracetamol for mild to moderate pain. They also reduce fever. In regular or higher doses NSAIDs have an additional anti-inflammatory action to reduce redness, stiffness and swelling. High doses are used to treat acute gout.

Although NSAIDs were widely prescribed to treat all types of arthritis, their use is now limited by their potential for side effects. These side effects range from gastric irritation to worsening existing asthma in some people. NSAIDs have also been associated with kidney and cardiovascular problems. As a result, you shouldn't take NSAIDs (except under supervision) if you have a history of peptic ulcers or asthma, or you are pregnant or breastfeeding. Check with a pharmacist for interactions if you are taking other drugs.

TOPICAL PAINKILLERS

These are painkillers that you can massage gently into the skin. Some topical painkillers – called rubefacients – contain substances that cause continuous, low-level stimulation of the skin bringing increased blood flow, warmth and redness. This helps to reduce the transmission of pain signals from the underlying joint. Rubefacients typically include substances such as menthol or methyl salicylate (oil of wintergreen), or capsaicin (from chilli peppers).

Some NSAIDs are also available in the form of topical creams or gels, which penetrate through the skin to the underlying joint to reduce pain and inflammation.

TRANSCUTANEOUS ELECTRICAL NERVE STIMULATION (TENS)

This is a drug-free way to relieve pain. A typical TENS machine contains four pads that are stuck to your back, or around a painful joint. The device then generates small pulses of electric current that stimulate your nerve endings. This sends pain-blocking signals to the brain and temporarily numbs surrounding tissues in a similar way to acupuncture.

CARTILAGE TRANSPLANTS

If you have osteoarthritis, cartilage cells can be harvested from one of your healthy joints, grown in the laboratory, and transplanted back into a joint whose cartilage is damaged. The chondrocytes (cartilage-making cells) then produce a healthy new joint lining, although it's not yet clear how long this new cartilage is likely to last.

CORTICOSTEROIDS

These are synthetic drug forms of the adrenal hormones that are involved in the body's response to stress. In nature, steroid hormones allow you to perform feats of endurance with little perception of pain. They have a powerful anti-inflammatory action to reduce pain and swelling. They can also damp down abnormal immune processes such as those involved in rheumatoid arthritis.

You can take corticosteroid drugs orally or have them injected directly into a joint. The long-term use of oral corticosteroids is limited by their potential side effects, which include bone thinning, glucose intolerance and weight gain. However, short, sharp oral courses (seven to 10 days) of a corticosteroid called prednisolone can provide considerable benefits with minimal risk of side effects. And some evidence suggests that low-dose prednisolone (7.5mg daily) can reduce the rate of joint destruction in early, moderate-to-severe rheumatoid arthritis if you take it for two to four years.

If you take oral corticosteroids for longer than three weeks, you are usually given a steroid treatment card that warns against stopping treatment suddenly – the dose should always be tapered off to allow recovery from any suppression of your adrenal glands.

Injections of corticosteroid drugs can reduce pain and inflammation, but repeated injections, especially into a weight-bearing joint such as the knee, can lead to joint degeneration. Most doctors prefer not to inject a joint more than three times.

OPIOID DRUGS

If you have severe joint pain, you may be prescribed stronger morphine-related painkillers, such as fentanyl or buprenorphine. They usually come in the form of skin patches that slowly release the drug into your circulation. Opiates have a direct action on pain perception in the brain. Other opiate-related drugs include codeine and dihydrocodeine. They work well in combination with paracetamol for occasional use when pain flares up, but they cause constipation if you use them regularly. They can also be addictive.

There is a wide range of other potential side effects associated with taking opiates. These include nausea, vomiting, drowsiness, headache, flushing, dizziness and palpitations. Patches may cause redness, rash or itching at the site of application.

DISEASE-MODIFYING ANTI-RHEUMATIC DRUGS (DMARDS)

DMARDs are a motley collection of unrelated drugs that interfere with different aspects of the immune response. They are prescribed as early as possible in autoimmune joint diseases such as rheumatoid arthritis,

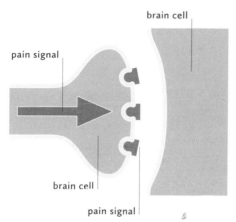

brain cell

pain signal

brain cell

pain signal

HOW OPIOID DRUGS RELIEVE PAIN
Opioid drugs both reduce the transmission of pain signals and affect the way pain is perceived. Although pain may still be present, it no longer seems to matter.

BEFORE TAKING OPIOID DRUG

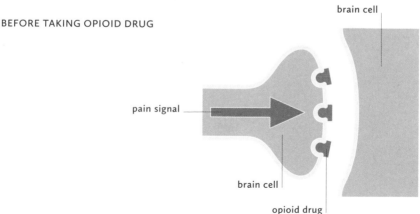

brain cell

pain signal

brain cell

opioid drug

AFTER TAKING OPIOID DRUG

psoriatic arthropathy and ankylosing spondylitis, as they may reduce the progressive destruction of inflamed joints.

The action of DMARDs isn't completely understood, but we know they affect white-blood-cell function to damp down abnormal immune reactions. It may take several weeks for DMARDs to produce an effect.

Drugs in this group include gold salts (sodium aurothiomalate and auranofin), penicillamine, leflunomide, sulfasalazine (an antibiotic), some anti-rejection drugs used in tissue transplants (azathioprine and ciclosporin), some anti-cancer drugs (methotrexate and cyclophosphamide), and some anti-malaria drugs (chloroquine and hydrochloroquine). The potential for side effects is high – you'll need regular checks to monitor your blood pressure, blood count, and liver and kidney function while taking DMARDs.

BIOLOGICAL RESPONSE MODIFIERS (BMRS)

If a DMARD has no effect on an autoimmune form of arthritis, doctors may recommend a BMR. These inhibit the production or action of cytokines (chemicals secreted by white blood cells during inflammation). BMRs are given by injection or by infusion – they can relieve rheumatoid arthritis, psoriatic arthropathy or ankylosing spondylitis in some people, but are stopped if there is no improvement within three months.

Because they reduce your immune response, BMRs increase the risk of serious infections such as tuberculosis, pneumonia and septicemia. Other potential side effects include nausea, headache, abdominal pain, allergic reactions, blood disorders and injection-site reactions. Because the potential for side effects is high, you usually have regular health checks while taking BMRs. You should tell your doctor if you are in contact with someone who has chickenpox or shingles.

OTHER DRUGS USED TO TREAT ARTHRITIS

If you have septic arthritis, you'll be treated with antimicrobial drugs, according to the bacteria, virus or fungus that's responsible for your infection. The usual cause is a bacterium, which is treatable by antibiotics such as oxacillin, nafcillin, vancomycin or cefotaxime. The septic joint is also drained. If your arthritis results from Lyme disease, tetracycline antibiotics can help.

A variety of medicines are used to treat gout (in addition to high doses of NSAIDs). Colchicine – a poison originally derived from the autumn crocus – reduces the pain and inflammation of gout, but is used only on a short-term basis because it has arsenic-like side effects such as vomiting and abdominal pain. It's often used to relieve gout symptoms as you begin longer-term treatment with allopurinol. This ensures that gout doesn't recur before allopurinol achieves its full effect. Allopurinol is used only after an acute attack has subsided as, paradoxically, it makes an acute attack worse. Side effects of allopurinol are rare, but may include rashes, allergic reactions, hepatitis and kidney problems. Another drug, sulfinpyrazone, can treat gout, but a potential side effect is the production of uric-acid kidney stones.

SURGERY

When pain and disability are severe enough to damage your quality of life, and drug treatment hasn't worked, your doctor may recommend surgery. Ninety percent of people undergoing joint replacement report rapid pain relief, improved mobility and better quality of life.

SYNOVECTOMY

This is the removal of the inflamed, thickened synovial membrane that can overgrow and invade the joint in rheumatoid arthritis. This procedure can improve joint mobility and reduce pain and inflammation. Depending on how much excess membrane needs to be removed, this procedure can occur through a small incision; during joint keyhole surgery (arthroscopy); or during an open operation in which the whole joint is exposed. The procedure can provide relief for one or more years and postpone the need for joint replacement.

OSTEOTOMY

This involves the removal of a section of bone to realign a joint and correct deformity. It can improve pain and mobility in osteoarthritic joints such as the knee, in vertebral joints stiffened by ankylosing spondylitis, and in joints, such as the hip, that are deformed by rheumatoid arthritis. It can take several months to recover from osteotomy, but the benefits usually last years. The procedure can make future joint replacement more difficult, because it alters your joint anatomy.

ARTHRODESIS

This is the removal or fusion of a joint so that your bones lock into place. The procedure stabilizes the joint and relieves pain in joints involving the vertebral column, thumb and wrist. Hip, knee and ankle joints can also be fused into a position that allows optimal function, so you can walk well, but with a limp. Weight-bearing joints are usually fused in cases where joint replacement is unsuitable; for example,

HIP REPLACEMENT
During hip replacement, part of your thigh bone is removed and replaced with a metal shaft and ball. The ball fits into a plastic socket that's inserted into your pelvis.

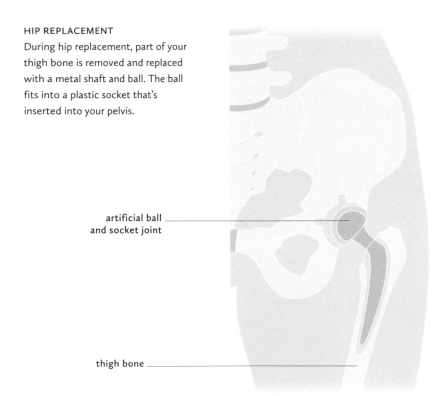

artificial ball and socket joint

thigh bone

because of osteoporosis or abnormal anatomy from a congenital dislocation of the hip or a deformed fracture.

ARTHROPLASTY

This is the replacement of damaged parts of a joint with a new, artificial prosthesis. The joints most usually replaced include the ankle, finger, hip, knee, elbow and shoulder. In most cases, the whole joint is replaced, with metal and plastic surfaces replacing all the bone and cartilage within a joint, while in others, just one part of the joint may need to be renewed, such as in hip resurfacing, where the ball-shaped head of the femur is preserved, reshaped and capped with a metal prosthesis.

You are encouraged to use a new joint soon after arthroplasty – often the next day. Ninety percent of people undergoing joint replacement report rapid pain relief, improved mobility and better quality of life.

PART TWO

THE NATURAL HEALTH APPROACH

The natural health approach to treating arthritis involves a number of complementary therapies that you can use in conjunction with the treatment your doctor prescribes. These include aromatherapy, herbal medicine, naturopathy, hydrotherapy, homeopathy and reflexology. I also take you through the principles of manipulation therapies, such as chiropractic and osteopathy, and explain how Eastern approaches, such as acupuncture, yoga and qigong, can help alleviate joint pain. Magnets and copper are very popular in the treatment of arthritis and I explain how you can put these to practical use. Tackling arthritis through the food you eat is important, too – by following a diet that is rich in antioxidants, and by avoiding foods that may act as a trigger for your arthritis, you can reduce the level of inflammation in your joints. Simple measures such as eating more fruit, vegetables and oily fish can go a long way to help. Some dietary supplements, such as glucosamine, are extremely beneficial. You may also find that lifestyle changes can provide symptom relief – I explain how you can start exercising in ways that won't hurt your joints, and how to reduce your weight if you need to – losing weight is a very effective way of relieving pressure on your joints.

COMPLEMENTARY APPROACHES TO TREATMENT

There are a number of therapies you can use to complement the orthodox treatment of arthritis. These include practitioner-led therapies, such as reiki, osteopathy and chiropractic, and approaches in which you will benefit from initial professional guidance, such as naturopathy and herbal medicine before continuing by yourself at home. Several self-help therapies are also beneficial, such as hydrotherapy, and magnetic and copper therapy.

Over the next few pages I explore the main complementary therapies that are used to treat all forms of arthritis. Some, such as aromatherapy, meditation and yoga, work mainly through relaxation, which reduces strain on muscles, ligaments and joints; while others, such as acupuncture, reflexology and homeopathy, harness your body's own natural healing abilities to reduce pain. In contrast, herbal medicine uses plant extracts that have a physiological effect on the body, modifying its function in a similar way to some prescribed anti-inflammatory drugs.

In many cases, complementary therapies can improve your symptoms enough to reduce your need to take orthodox painkillers. This is important because some painkillers, such as non-steroidal anti-inflammatory drugs (NSAIDs), are associated with a number of adverse side effects (see pages 28–29).

CHECK THERAPISTS' CREDENTIALS

If you choose to visit a therapist, it's important to consult someone who has the appropriate credentials. Ask a potential therapist about his or her qualifications, and experience and successes in treating arthritis. Make sure the therapist is accredited with the appropriate umbrella organization; and check he or she carries indemnity insurance. Alternatively, look for a therapist via an umbrella organization – most will send you a list of their qualified practitioners. Many organizations also have a facility on their website to help you find a therapist in your area. Some useful contact details are provided in the resource section of this book (see pages 234–235).

CONSULTING A THERAPIST

Having checked the qualifications of your chosen therapist (see box on the opposite page), you should find out how long your course of treatment is likely to last, and how much it's likely to cost, before commiting yourself to an appointment. Having received some guidance from a therapist, you may find you need only one or two consultations before you can treat yourself at home. For example, if you visit a homeopath or an aromatherapist, you can simply carry on taking the remedies they prescribe for you or, in the case of aromatherapy, experiment with your own essential-oil blends. Other therapies, particularly those that rely on hands-on treatments, such as reflexology, massage, chiropractic and osteopathy, require you to attend regular appointments so that you continue to experience benefits.

AROMATHERAPY

Aromatherapy is one of the most popular complementary therapies for arthritis. The aromatic essential oils produced by the leaves, stems, bark, flowers, roots or seeds of many plants have a natural, painkilling action or a muscle-relaxant effect to reduce spasms. As essential oils are highly concentrated, you must first dilute them with a carrier oil such as almond, avocado, calendula, grapeseed, jojoba or wheatgerm oil before putting them on your skin.

USEFUL ESSENTIAL OILS

If you have osteoarthritis, any of the following essential oils may help: basil, black pepper, coriander, ginger, lemon, marjoram, peppermint and thyme. If you have autoimmune arthritis (for example, rheumatoid or psoriatic arthritis), choose from any of these essential oils: benzoin, camomile (German and Roman), eucalyptus, peppermint, geranium, lavender, lemon, rosemary and thyme.

The following blend is useful for all types of arthritis (and can also help to reduce depression): eight drops each of eucalyptus and lavender oil mixed with four drops each of marjoram oil, peppermint oil and rosemary oil. Mix this blend with 100ml carrier oil (blended from 45ml almond oil, 45ml apricot oil and 10ml jojoba oil). A lavender and rosemary oil blend (diluted with a carrier oil) may also be helpful.

HOW TO USE ESSENTIAL OILS

Essential oils can be inhaled from a tissue or diffused into the atmosphere using a candle-lit burner, but your joints will benefit most from the direct methods of application described below. If you apply heat to your joint (by using a hot compress or during a hot bath), it's important to move the joint as much as possible immediately afterward. This will help you derive maximum benefits from the heat treatment, and it will also prevent congestion, which may make joint stiffness worse.

MASSAGE OIL

To make a massage oil, add one to three drops of your chosen essential-oil blend to 5ml carrier oil. For a larger quantity add 30 to 40 drops to 100ml carrier oil. Massage into painful joints.

AROMATHERAPY BATH

Add five drops of essential oil/s to 15ml carrier oil and mix. Draw your

---

USE ESSENTIAL OILS WITH CAUTION
- Don't take essential oils internally.
- Before using an essential oil blend, put a small amount on a patch of skin and leave it for at least an hour to check it doesn't cause an adverse reaction.
- Don't use essential oils if you have high blood pressure or epilepsy, or if you are pregnant (or likely to be), except under supervision.
- Don't use undiluted oils on your skin.
- Keep essential oils away from the eyes.
- Essential oils are flammable, so don't put them on an open flame.

bath so that it's comfortably hot, then add the oil mix. Close the bathroom door to keep in the vapours and soak for 15 to 20 minutes, preferably in candlelight.

HOT COMPRESS

Fill a medium-size bowl with comfortably hot water and add six drops of your chosen essential oil/s. Fold a piece of clean, cotton cloth and dip it into the bowl. Squeeze out some of the excess water, but not too much. Place the hot, wet cloth over the painful joint until it cools down to body temperature. Repeat this two or three times.

HERBAL MEDICINE

Herbalism is one of the most effective complementary therapies for treating arthritis. Herbalists use different parts of different plants, depending on which has the highest concentration of active ingredients.

HERBAL TREATMENTS

Herbal treatments for arthritis are best prescribed by a medical herbalist. Some products may not be available over the counter, but if you do choose to buy your own, select those that have been "standardized" – this means the remedy contains a consistent amount of active ingredient so each dose provides the same pain-relieving or anti-inflammatory benefits.

ARNICA (*ARNICA MONTANA*)

Herbalists use this mountain flower to make a topical gel. Research shows that it's as effective as ibuprofen gel for treating painful joints.
Typical use: apply it two to four times a day.

BROMELAIN

This enzyme from pineapple stems has an anti-inflammatory action. It can significantly reduce acute knee pain, stiffness and swelling associated with osteoarthritis and rheumatoid arthritis. It can also reduce pain and

bruising after surgery (consult your surgeon if you'd like to try it). Avoid it if you are taking blood-thinning medication, such as aspirin or warfarin.
Typical dose: 250–500mg three times a day. Select supplements with at least 2,000 milk-clotting units.

DEVIL'S CLAW (*HARPAGOPHYTUM PROCUMBENS*)
This eases pain and is as effective as a non-steroidal, anti-inflammatory drug (NSAID). Avoid it if you have peptic ulcers or indigestion.
Typical dose: 1–10g daily (depending on concentration of extract – to provide around 50mg harpagoside daily).

FRANKINCENSE (*BOSWELLIA DALZIELII*)
This contains anti-inflammatory substances called boswellic acids, which are as effective at relieving pain as many NSAIDs.
Typical dose: 200–400mg two or three times a day, standardized for at least 37.5 percent boswellic acids.

GINGER (*ZINGIBER OFFICINALE*)
This relieves joint pain by suppressing the release of inflammatory chemicals. It has a cartilage-protecting action and eases the pain of knee osteoarthritis on standing and after walking.
Typical dose: powdered ginger root standardized for 0.4 percent volatile oils; 250mg two to four times daily.

OLIVE (*OLEA EUROPAEA*)
Olive leaf extracts contain anti-inflammatory antioxidants that can decrease pain in people with osteoarthritis, and reduce inflammation in people with rheumatoid arthritis.
Typical dose: 400mg a day.

ROSEHIP (*ROSA CANINA*)
The extracts can reduce the pain and stiffness associated with rheumatoid and osteoarthritis by more than 80 percent.
Typical dose: 2.5g once or twice a day.

TURMERIC (*CURCUMA LONGA*)

Often used in Indian cooking, this root contains an active ingredient, curcumin, that has a powerful anti-inflammatory action equivalent to that of some prescribed corticosteroids.

Typical dose: 500–1200mg once a day, standardized to 95 percent curcuminoids.

WHITE WILLOW (*SALIX ALBA*)

The bark of the white willow contains salicylic acid – the parent compound from which aspirin is synthesized. Although slower acting, white willow offers pain-relieving properties similar to aspirin, but with less risk of stomach irritation. Avoid if you have peptic ulcers, asthma or are sensitive to aspirin.

Typical dose: 150–300mg every six hours.

NATUROPATHY

Naturopathy employs a range of therapies that help you to maintain a healthy balance between your body's biochemistry and structure, and your emotions. The theory that underpins naturopathy is that once your body and mind are in a state of equilibrium, they are able to heal themselves. A naturopath uses a variety of complementary approaches, including nutritional medicine, herbal remedies, hydrotherapy, massage, homeopathy, reflexology, relaxation techniques, hypnotherapy and yoga. Many naturopaths are also trained in osteopathy or chiropractic manipulation.

HEALTHY DIET AND LIFESTYLE

The goal of naturopathy is to identify and treat the cause of a disease rather than to suppress the symptoms. In the case of arthritis, naturopaths believe that an accumulation of toxic acids in the joints is responsible. They recommend that you reduce your intake of highly refined, processed foods, saturated animal fats, sugar and salt; eat more fruit, vegetables and

BEE VENOM THERAPY

Some naturopaths use bee venom to treat arthritis. Bee venom contains a mix of chemicals that, paradoxically, can relieve joint and muscle pain in arthritic and rheumatic conditions. The venom is harvested using a mild electro-stimulant technique that doesn't harm the bees. Treatment is via either injections combined with local anesthetic – typically into acupuncture points – or a topical balm. The balm often contains other natural ingredients such as capsaicin (from chilli peppers) and tea tree oil. When applied to a painful joint twice a day, the balm stimulates the release of cortisol – one of the body's most powerful, natural anti-inflammatory hormones – and has an analgesic, anti-inflammatory and immune-boosting effect. When given by injection, you will experience stinging, swelling and aching for several hours. Avoid bee venom therapy if you're allergic to bee stings, or have health problems, such as high blood pressure.

wholegrains; and make sure that you are taking on sufficient water. Other advice might include avoiding certain foods, for example, foods from the nightshade family such as tomatoes, aubergines and peppers (see pages 77–78), red meat (see pages 79), or dairy products. You may be advised to follow an alkaline diet (see pages 79–81). A naturopath is also likely to recommend supplements such as omega-3 fish oils, glucosamine, chondroitin, MSM, calcium, magnesium, copper, and the herbs and spices ginger, frankincense and Devil's claw. You can use fresh ginger to make a healing tea.

Apart from dietary treatment a naturopath may offer hydrotherapy treatments, plus advice on getting plenty of sleep, taking regular exercise and finding ways to relax. There's an emphasis in naturopathy on the importance of fresh air, sunshine, a clean environment, a stress-free lifestyle and a positive mental attitude.

HYDROTHERAPY

Hydrotherapy uses water as a healing substance, whether in the form of hot or cold liquid, steam or ice. Temperature plays an important role in hydrotherapy, as both heat and cold have analgesic effects. Cold baths stimulate the metabolism and help to reduce or prevent swelling and inflammation by constricting blood vessels. Warm water at body temperature is used to reduce sensory perception in floatation therapy; and hot water boosts circulation, helps muscles relax, eases aching joints and reduces stiffness. Some treatments use hot and cold water alternately to reduce muscle spasm and boost production of the anti-inflammatory hormone cortisone.

Researchers have found that having a warm bath plus an ice massage can significantly raise pain thresholds in people with rheumatoid arthritis – the effect occurs immediately. They found that cryotherapy (application of ice) alone also has an immediate effect on pain threshold and lasts for 30 minutes. In people with osteoarthritis of the knee, having a 20-minute ice massage, five days a week for three weeks improves the strength of the quadriceps muscle by around 30 percent, and the range of knee flexion by eight percent. Another study showed that cold packs effectively reduce knee swelling.

HYDROTHERAPY TECHNIQUES

Hydrotherapy uses a variety of different techniques, including bathing in mineral solutions, seaweed extracts (thalassotherapy), mud, peat, spa waters or sea water, and swimming in a pool. Therapists may also recommend a sitz bath (in which you immerse your buttocks, thighs and lower back in water), saunas, steam rooms, whirlpools, hot tubs, high-pressure jets, hot compresses, wraps, ice packs and aromatherapy baths. All can ease the pain of arthritis.

EXERCISING IN WATER

Hospital physiotherapy departments often offer exercise sessions in a warm swimming pool (typically at a temperature of 33–37°C/ 91.4–98.6°F). The warmth relaxes your muscles, and the buoyancy of the water reduces your body weight by 85 percent, which takes pressure off your joints making it easier to exercise. Moving your arms and legs against the water also offers enough resistance to help improve muscle

SELF-HELP HYDROTHERAPY

You can recreate some of the effects of floatation therapy (see opposite page) at home using mineral salts from the Dead Sea (available from larger health-food stores and pharmacies). Add a small sachet (250g/9oz) of Dead Sea salts to a warm bath and relax for 20 minutes (making sure not to get the water in your eyes). Then wrap yourself in a warm towel and lie down in a warm room. Another useful hydrotherapy technique is to exercise your hands in a bowl of hot soapy water – open and close your hands and wriggle your fingers until they start to loosen up. Do this every morning to ease stiffness at the start of the day. Taking a hot bath or shower during the day can also ease pains and help maintain your mobility. If you find it difficult getting in and out of the bath, consider investing in grab rails, a bath lift or a walk-in bath.

strength. This kind of exercise is beneficial for people with all types of arthritis, but people with rheumatoid arthritis find it particularly beneficial. When 115 people with rheumatoid arthritis received either weekly 30-minute sessions of hydrotherapy or similar exercises on land, 87 percent of those treated with hydrotherapy reported they were "much better" or "very much better", compared with only 48 percent of those treated with land exercise.

HOT AND COLD PACKS

A therapist may recommend that you use hot and cold gel-packs to ease joint pain and stiffness – you put the packs in either the microwave or the freezer. Some commercially available heat pads also contain magnets for additional benefits (see pages 51–52). If you don't have a gel-pack, a bag of frozen peas can work as well – it readily moulds to the shape of an affected joint. My guidelines for when to use ice and when to use heat are as follows:

- If your joint is swollen and painful, use an ice pack.
- If your joint is stiff, but not swollen, use a heat pack.
- If you have an acute injury (one that happened within the last six weeks) use an ice pack.

- If in doubt, use ice first. If this isn't as effective as you would like, try a heat pack instead.

When using an ice pack, take care to avoid freezer burn. Instead of applying an ice pack directly to your skin, wrap it in a cloth, and apply for up to 10 minutes at a time – remove for a few minutes then re-apply.

FLOATATION THERAPY

This involves lying in a light-proof, sound-insulated tank that contains a shallow, super-saturated solution of Epsom salts (magnesium sulphate). The minerals neutralize many of the effects of gravity, which helps you to relax completely both physically and mentally – it's estimated that 90 percent of all brain activity is concerned with the effects of gravitational pull on the body (for example, correcting posture and maintaining balance). The temperature of the floatation water is a constant 34.5°C/93.5°F (skin temperature).

You must be relatively mobile to have floatation therapy as you need to climb safely in and out of the tank, which resembles an enclosed bath. Most people float naked, but you can wear a bathing costume if you prefer. Many large towns contain a floatation centre. For best results, try a course of five weekly floats.

HOW FLOATATION THERAPY WORKS

The tank screens out light and sound so your brain is cut off from virtually all external stimulation.

- This induces a profoundly relaxed state in which you generate the special brainwaves – theta waves – associated with meditation, creative thought and feelings of serenity. There's a significant increase in the secretion of endorphins – your brain's natural painkillers.
- As well as relieving chronic pain, endorphins produce feelings of euphoria and improve the quality of your sleep.
- The benefits last for up to three weeks. (In addition to easing arthritis symptoms, floatation therapy can lower high blood pressure.)

HOMEOPATHY

Homeopathy is based on the concept that like cures like – tiny amounts of a potential toxin can treat symptoms similar to those it would produce if used at full strength. Clinical trials show that homeopathy is significantly better than a placebo at treating arthritis.

VISITING A HOMEOPATH

A homeopath prescribes treatments according to your symptoms, personality, lifestyle, likes and dislikes, as well as your constitutional type. He or she will usually prescribe a 6c or 12c potency at first, followed by a higher potency (30c) if you experience partial symptom relief combined with a return of symptoms when you stop taking the remedy.

Take homeopathic remedies on their own without eating or drinking for at least 30 minutes before or afterward. If your symptoms worsen initially, persevere with treatment – it's a sign that a remedy is working. If there's no improvement after taking a remedy for the allotted time, consult your homeopath.

COPPER THERAPY

When you wear copper jewelry, trace amounts of copper are absorbed through your skin. Many people find this is effective at easing their joint symptoms. It still isn't known exactly how copper exerts its therapeutic effect, but it's known that copper is involved in the synthesis of collagen – a major structural protein in bones and joints – and it's thought that a lack of copper contributes to the development of inflammatory diseases. As well as being important for joint health, copper may have a direct analgesic effect.

HOW TO USE COPPER

Although you can get copper from your diet, the amounts present in food are tiny and only a relatively small proportion of the mineral is actually

HOMEOPATHIC REMEDIES FOR ARTHRITIS

These remedies are often prescribed for people with arthritis, but a homeopath may prescribe others depending on your symptoms and your constitutional type.

REMEDY	PREPARED FROM	USED TO TREAT
Arnica	Leopard's bane/sneezewort	Arthritis in a joint previously damaged by trauma.
Apis	Honey bee	Hot, swollen, painful, stiff joints, especially the fingers and ankles.
Belladonna	Deadly nightshade	Septic arthritis with a hot, red, tender joint, plus fever.
Calcarea phosphorica	Calcium phosphate	Weakness and pain in the hips.
Colchicum	Meadow saffron	Gout with a red, hot, swollen, excruciatingly painful joint.
Kali iodatum	Potassium iodide	Swollen, painful knee joints, with symptoms worse at night and in damp weather.
Ledum	Wild rosemary/marsh tea	Arthritis that starts in the lower limbs and moves to joints in the upper body.
Lycopodium	Club moss	Recurrent attacks of gout in someone with arthritis in other joints, and frequent cramps.
Rhus toxicodendron	Poison ivy	Swollen, stiff joints that are initially painful then eased by movement.
Sabina	Juniper	Arthritis with red, shiny, swollen joints.
Urtica	Stinging nettle	Gout with stinging pains and itchiness.

absorbed. Foods with the highest copper concentrations include kidney, shellfish, nuts, seeds, pulses and wholegrains, and vegetables that have been grown in copper-rich soil. It's thought that average copper intakes are around 1.6mg a day, but, of this, 70 percent isn't absorbed by the gut because copper becomes bound to other bowel contents such as sugars, sweeteners and refined flour.

Copper is much more readily absorbed through the skin. However, wearing copper products doesn't help everyone with arthritis. The effectiveness of a copper product is thought to depend on the level of copper already present in your body – if you are copper-deficient, you may benefit; but if your levels are already adequate, copper products may not help.

In order for copper to work properly you need to have adequate levels of zinc in your body. The ideal dietary ratio of copper to zinc is one to 10. I recommend that you obtain at least 15mg of zinc a day from your diet or that you take zinc supplements. Zinc is found in seafood, particularly oysters. Even if you don't use copper products, zinc is a useful mineral for people with rheumatoid arthritis (see page 90).

COPPER JEWELRY
When you wear copper jewelry such as bracelets or rings, copper is absorbed through the skin at an estimated rate of 100–150mg copper a year. In one study of more than 300 people with a variety of types of arthritis, copper bracelets worn on the wrists and ankles were analyzed to see how much copper they lost over a period of 50 days. Results showed

COPPER SHOE INSERTS
Try wearing shoe inserts made from copper. The inserts, developed by a podiatrist, are called "Copper Heelers" (see page 214) and they fit easily into your shoes. It's thought that acid sweat from your feet hastens the absorption of copper through your soles. Anecdotal evidence suggests that the product significantly reduces joint pain.

that they lost between 80 and 90mg. Participants in the study reported positive benefits as a result of wearing the bracelets. Interestingly, some other participants in the study, who wore a placebo bracelet (having previously worn an authentic copper one), experienced a significant deterioration in their arthritis symptoms. In another trial involving 240 people with rheumatoid arthritis, those wearing copper bracelets experienced a statistically significant reduction in their arthritis symptoms when compared with participants wearing a placebo bracelet.

Expect a slight green discoloration of your skin when you wear copper jewelry – it's caused by the interaction of copper and sweat.

MAGNETIC THERAPY

Applying a magnet to an arthritic joint can help in a number of ways. First, it encourages small blood vessels to dilate and causes iron-containing red blood cells to line up in the same direction so they can pass through blood capillaries more easily. This increases blood flow to the affected joint.

Second, magnetized red blood cells are able to carry oxygen more efficiently, so the joint receives more oxygen and nutrients, and toxins are removed more easily. Finally, magnets help to damp down inflammation and pain, and they stimulate the production of the body's natural painkillers (endorphins). Research shows that exposure to a static magnet can increase endorphin levels by 25 percent within one hour and by 45 percent within two hours.

A study in Japan involving 121 patients with severe, chronic shoulder pain revealed that 82 percent of those using high-strength magnets showed significant improvement within four days. In those treated with low-strength magnets, there was only a 37-percent improvement rate.

USING MAGNETS THERAPEUTICALLY
Therapeutic magnets are widely used to alleviate the pain of arthritis and other inflammatory conditions. They often take the form of jewelry or

WHEN TO AVOID MAGNETIC THERAPY

Although magnetic therapy can alleviate arthritis symptoms, there are certain considerations to be aware of. Keep magnets away from computer disks and other magnetic media. Do not use magnets:

- If you have an infection.
- If you have recently had chicken pox.
- On open wounds (except under medical supervision).
- If you have hemophilia.
- If you have a heart pacemaker.
- If you are undergoing dialysis.
- If you are using an insulin pump or drug patch (use magnets only under medical supervision).
- If you have a surgically implanted metal screw in your body.
- If you are pregnant or trying to conceive.

shoe in-soles. You can also buy magnetic wraps to wrap around joints such as the knee, ankle or elbow – the wraps are secured with Velcro and they don't restrict your movement. As well as providing magnetic therapy they also give support to a painful joint. Adhesive magnetic patches are available, too – you can use patches in the following ways:

- Stick them over acupuncture points near the site of pain. Consult an acupuncturist for advice.
- Stick the patches directly on any areas of tenderness.
- Stick several patches on the skin so that they surround the painful joint.

When buying a magnet, choose one that's strong enough to have a therapeutic effect. The strength of a magnetic field is measured in units known as teslas or gauss. One tesla is equivalent to 10,000 gauss. Magnets that are used for healing have field strengths that range from 200–2000 gauss (20 to 200 milliteslas). For optimum effect, I suggest you select a therapeutic magnet with a field strength of at least 500 gauss.

MASSAGE

As well as encouraging general relaxation, massage eases muscle tension and stimulates the release of endorphins – the body's natural painkillers. People with all forms of arthritis can benefit from regular massage.

VISITING A MASSAGE THERAPIST

During a massage, you usually lie on a massage table with a hole over which you rest your head. Alternatively, you may sit, leaning forward in a massage chair, or lie on a pad on the floor. The part of the body to be massaged is usually uncovered, but you can wear clothes during some techniques, such as acupressure, shiatsu, tui na and Thai massage.

TYPES OF MASSAGE

A massage therapist uses a variety of strokes to stimulate the soft tissues; for example, rubbing, drumming, kneading, wringing, friction and applying deep pressure. More than 100 different types of massage are recognized. Any of the following types may help relieve your symptoms – tell your massage therapist prior to a massage that you have arthritis.

SWEDISH MASSAGE

A therapist uses massage oil and lotion. Strokes are long, smooth and gentle.

AROMATHERAPY MASSAGE

This combines Swedish massage with essential oils selected for your particular joint symptoms (see pages 39–41).

AYURVEDIC MASSAGE

One or more therapists rub warm, herb-infused medicinal oil into every part of your body, including your scalp.

BOWEN TECHNIQUE

This uses rolling movements over muscles, ligaments, tendons and joints.

DEEP TISSUE MASSAGE

This focuses on a specific joint, muscle or muscle group. Therapists use their fingers, knuckles, elbows and thumbs, and the heel of the hand and even the foot to massage deeper into a problem area, ease muscle spasm and improve movement and mobility.

HOT STONE MASSAGE

This form of massage involves therapists warming smooth stones (such as basalt or marble) in water, then coating them in oil and using them to massage and relax your muscles.

MYOFASCIAL RELEASE

This stretches the tissue layer (fascia) that binds muscles together, allowing them to move more freely.

SHIATSU

This is a Japanese form of massage in which practitioners use their fingers and thumbs to massage and stimulate acupressure points on the skin. Each point is held for a few seconds.

THAI MASSAGE

More energetic than other forms, Thai massage involves stretching your body into a series of yoga-like postures. The practitioner uses their hands, forearms and feet to apply firm, rhythmic pressure, including pulling fingers, toes and ears.

TUI NA

This is a form of Chinese massage in which muscles are pushed, pulled, stretched and kneaded.

ROLFING

Also known as structural integration, this combines massage with deep pressure and postural adjustments in which the therapist slowly stretches and repositions your body's supportive soft tissues.

CRANIAL OSTEOPATHY

This branch of osteopathy evolved from the understanding that the fused joints of the skull retain slight flexibility, so the head becomes slightly wider from side to side, and slightly shorter from front to back, when breathing in. Cranial osteopaths believe this happens to accommodate natural movements within the cerebrospinal fluid (CSF) that bathes and nourishes the brain and spinal cord, which is said to pulsate at six to 15 times per minute. Practitioners sense this pulsation (known as the cranial rhythmic impulse) with their hands and "listen" to the inner movements and tensions inside the patient. They use their highly trained sense of touch to identify disturbances in the joints of the skull, which are then manipulated using gentle but specific adjustments to improve the circulation of CSF, blood and lymph in the head. The technique is gentle enough to use on newborn babies, and can help a wide range of conditions, including back and neck pain, especially for severe problems where a doctor has advised against direct spinal manipulation.

HELLERWORK

This is a modern adaptation of Rolfing in which massage and postural adjustments are combined with exploration of the emotions triggered by the release of tension.

OSTEOPATHY

Osteopathy involves gentle manipulation of the muscles, ligaments and joints to help relax muscles, correct poor alignment and reduce pain.

Osteopathy can help to treat all types of arthritis, and is effective at reducing pain, especially in the neck, lower back and hip. It can also reduce early morning stiffness and joint swelling, and improve joint movement and mobility. In fact, research suggests that, for treating back pain, spinal manipulation is more effective than either painkillers or exercise, with most people reporting striking benefits. A study published in the *New England Journal of Medicine* in 1999 found that osteopathic manipulation is as effective as standard medical care with painkillers, application of heat and cold and the use of a TENS machine (see page 29). On average, people receiving osteopathy were found to have achieved a 30-percent reduction in the level of their pain. Half as many people with arthritis who received osteopathic treatment needed NSAIDs compared with those on standard care (24 percent versus 54 percent).

VISITING AN OSTEOPATH

An osteopath will ask questions about your medical history, your general health and the specific problems you're experiencing at the moment. He or she will then assess the range of movement in your joints, and palpate (feel) parts of your body to detect areas of weakness, misalignment and excessive strain. The osteopath will also check your posture for symmetry and alignment of the pelvis, and compare the length of your legs. He or she will gently tap on muscle tendons at your knees, ankles, elbows and/ or wrists to test your nerve reflexes. If necessary, you may have further investigations, such as x-rays or blood tests.

Having got a full picture of your joint health, an osteopath will tailor a treatment plan to your needs. Osteopathic treatment involves manual manipulations that include gentle massage to relax tension, mobilization of stiff joints by stretching them rhythmically within their normal range of movement, and swift, high-velocity thrusts to correct poor bone alignments. Spinal manipulation may sometimes involve using your limbs to make levered thrusts. An osteopath may also give you advice on posture and how to reduce strain when lifting. He or she may recommend wearing flat shoes and using ergonomic aids when sitting and working at a desk and computer.

CHIROPRACTIC

Chiropractors specialize in the prevention, diagnosis and treatment of mechanical disorders of the muscles and joints, and their adverse effects on the nervous system. They mainly focus on misalignments of the spinal vertebrae, known as subluxations, which are common in people with arthritis. These misalignments can pinch or stretch tiny nerves to cause pain and reduce mobility. Chiropractors use their hands to manipulate the spinal column and the joints in which movement is restricted.

Research has shown that combining chiropractic spinal manipulation with the application of moist heat (see pages 46–47) is more effective in treating low-back pain caused by osteoarthritis than using heat alone. Chiropractic manipulation has also been shown to reduce pain in ankylosing spondylitis (see page 18) even where the sacroiliac joints and lumbar and cervical vertebrae are fused.

VISITING A CHIROPRACTOR

A chiropractor asks questions about your medical history, lifestyle, diet, exercise patterns, work, current symptoms and the type of bed on which you sleep. He or she will observe your posture when you stand and walk, and will ask how you sit at a desk. During the examination you are asked to variously stand, or sit or lie on a chiropractic couch, and you will be manoeuvred into a number of positions to assess your mobility and flexibility. This process, known as "motion palpation", helps the chiropractor assess which joints are moving freely, and which are stiff or locked. Motion palpation can identify the exact source of any pain that is troubling you. Irritation of a nerve in one area can sometimes lead to symptoms of discomfort in other parts of the body (known as referred pain), so manipulation may not be carried out at the site of your pain. For example, tingling in the fingers often results from misalignment

CRANIOSACRAL THERAPY

This involves the gentle manipulation of both the skull and the base of the spine. Craniosacral therapists believe the cranial rhythmic impulse (see box on page 36) affects every cell in the body. By gently manipulating and pressing on the head and sacrum, the therapist helps to achieve an even flow of the cranial rhythmic impulse, and facilitates the release of inner tensions over a wide area. Craniosacral therapy is used by many chiropractors – and osteopaths – to improve problems such as back and neck pain, headache, insomnia and stress.

(subluxation) of neck bones. A chiropractor may use other diagnostic tests such as x-rays, blood and urine tests and MRI scans.

Your treatment will consist of rapid, direct, yet gentle thrusts to correct vertebral subluxations. This helps bones to move into their correct positions, often with a click. This re-aligns muscles, tendons, ligaments and joints and helps to relieve pain and tension. Sometimes, a rubber-tipped instrument known as an "activator" is used to gently manipulate the vertebrae using small, precise, measured thrusts. Chiropractic also includes stretching and massage if appropriate.

McTimoney chiropractic is similar to standard chiropractic in that it focuses on the spine and nervous system, but also considers joints in other parts of the body. During a session, a McTimoney chiropractor will use his or her hands to check and adjust the spine, pelvis, chest, limbs and skull. He or she will use a number of light, swift hand movements including gentle fingertip manipulation to realign joints.

REFLEXOLOGY

Reflexology is an ancient technique that's at least 5,000 years old, and is based on similar principles to acupressure. It involves the stimulation and massage of points, known as reflexes, on the feet and hands. Each reflex corresponds to a specific part of the body – in such a way as to form a map of the body on the hands and feet. Look at the "maps" of the hands (opposite) to see where specific areas are represented. For example, areas on your palms (and the soles of your feet) relate to your shoulders, sciatic nerves and spine, while reflexes on the backs of your hands (and the tops of your feet) relate to your hips, knees, elbows and sacroiliac joints. Reflexology may help to reduce inflammation, relieve the symptoms of stress, and improve joint mobility and general well-being.

VISITING A REFLEXOLOGIST
During a reflexology session, a therapist massages all areas of your feet and/or hands using firm thumb and finger pressure. The therapist will

REFLEXOLOGY HAND MAPS

These maps show where specific areas of the body are represented on the fronts and backs of both hands. Massaging the areas that correspond to painful joints can help to relieve arthritis symptoms.

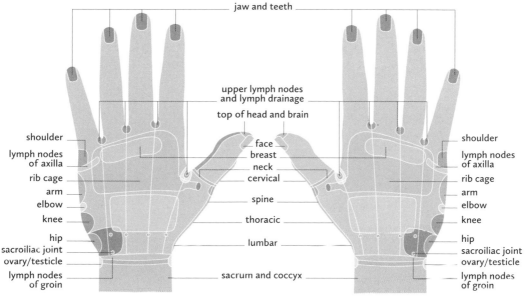

BACK OF LEFT HAND   BACK OF RIGHT HAND

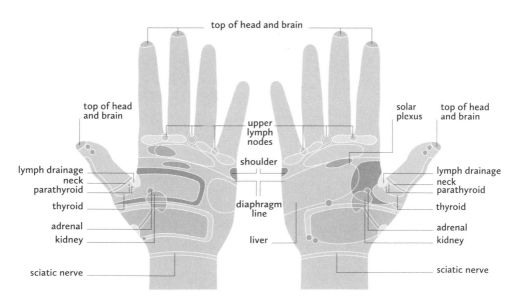

FRONT OF LEFT HAND   FRONT OF RIGHT HAND

SELF-HELP REFLEXOLOGY

You can help to ease your arthritis symptoms by gently massaging the knee, hip and spinal reflexes on your hands. Your spinal reflexes run along the sides of your thumbs, with the cervical area starting level with the base of your nails, followed by the thoracic spine, then the lumbar region in the curve where your hands and wrists meet, then the sacrum and coccyx at the sides of your wrists. Feel along these areas and stop on any that are tender. Press the reflexes, gradually pushing harder (up to the limit of comfort). Maintain the pressure for at least 20 seconds, then press and release in quick pulses of one or two seconds. Do this twice a day, morning and evening.

then treat specific problems such as arthritis by applying pressure and massaging the reflex points that correspond to the affected area. This stimulates nerve endings that pass from the hands or feet to the brain and out to the related part of the body – this helps to reduce symptoms such as pain, swelling and stiffness. The therapist may also massage reflexes corresponding to your adrenal glands to stimulate production of the anti-inflammatory hormone cortisone.

Full treatment usually lasts for 45 to 60 minutes and at the end of each session you will feel warm, contented and relaxed. For optimum benefit, book yourself in for one session a week for two months, then decide whether you find the treatment helps your arthritis. I have included details of reflexology organizations in the resources section at the end of this book (see page 235).

YOGA

Yoga, the ancient Eastern practice of movement, breathing and meditation, is beneficial for arthritis because it improves muscle strength, suppleness and range of movement. It also helps you to relax and manage pain. As well as the physical benefits, people who practise yoga regularly tend to enjoy feelings of emotional well-being and positivity – this can help you to cope with the challenge of living with arthritis.

STARTING YOGA

Yoga is best practised daily, but practising a few times a week for 30 to 60 minutes per session will also be beneficial. Join a beginner's class and tell your yoga teacher that you have arthritis. Once you've learned the basic postures and breathing techniques from a teacher, yoga is an excellent self-help therapy that you can continue at home. Gradually build up your practice time over a period of weeks and months.

Don't push yourself beyond your limits in yoga – learn to recognize the difference between the mild discomfort of stretching a muscle and the "bad" pain that comes from putting undue pressure on a joint.

Yoga is widely taught in the West – classes are held in sport and leisure centres, complementary health centres and dedicated yoga centres.

TYPES OF YOGA

There are many types of yoga ranging from the strenuous (ashtanga yoga) to the gentle (viniyoga). I suggest you try any of following three types – they are the most suitable for people with arthritis.

HATHA YOGA

This is the most popular form of yoga in the West. It involves a series of simple poses that flow comfortably from one to another at your own pace. Hatha yoga can improve hand-grip strength, reduce joint tenderness and improve the range of finger movement in people with either rheumatoid arthritis or osteoarthritis of the hands. Even people with severe rheumatoid arthritis can benefit. Research shows that twice weekly hour-long hatha yoga sessions can ease chronic low-back pain and improve balance and flexibility, with the benefits lasting for several months.

IYENGAR YOGA

This is a form of hatha yoga that's ideal if you have reduced flexibility. It employs items such as chairs, blocks and pillows to provide stability between your body and the floor if you're unable to bend fully into the postures. It's sometimes described as "meditation in action" as it focuses on symmetry, alignment and meditation, with postures being held for longer periods than in most other forms of yoga. Research shows that performing Iyengar yoga postures for 90 minutes once a week for eight weeks can reduce pain and stiffness and improve joint function in people with osteoarthritis of the knee. Iyengar yoga can also alleviate chronic low-back pain, reducing disability and use of pain medication.

VINIYOGA

This is also good for people with arthritis as its slow, gentle movements don't stress the joints. Viniyoga uses breath awareness, relaxation, meditation and guided imagery to reduce pain.

QIGONG

Qigong (pronounced "chee gong") is a traditional Chinese healing art that's sometimes referred to as "Chinese yoga" or "acupuncture without needles". It involves the use of gentle movements, stretches, guided imagery, and meditation to help you relax and breathe in a way that heals and nourishes the body. The basic postures of qigong are easy to learn and may be performed in any order. Qigong helps to strengthen your muscles and make you more supple. It also promotes feelings of lightness and calm that can help to improve your pain thresholds and help you live with arthritis on a day-to-day level.

Qigong is part of Traditional Chinese Medicine (TCM), which is based upon the belief that life-force energy, or qi, circulates throughout the body in channels known as meridians (see the illustrations on pages 64–65). Strengthening or balancing the flow of qi by practising qigong (or by having acupressure or acupuncture) improves your health and reduces your susceptibility to disease. In China, qigong is widely used to treat arthritis, which is believed to result from the body being invaded by a type of qi called "wind-cold-damp qi", which causes a qi blockage in certain joints. Treatment, therefore, involves eradicating the wind-cold-damp qi, eliminating the qi blockage in the affected joint, and introducing healthy and balanced qi into the area.

QIGONG WALKING

Particularly beneficial for arthritis, qigong walking uses more muscles than conventional walking. It encourages you to walk purposefully and slowly, and to move your arms as well as your legs in a smooth, relaxed rhythm. To practise qigong walking, bend your right arm and bring your right hand up to chest level (palm facing down, fingers naturally coiled in) as your left leg moves forward. Then swing your right arm down and back as you bring your left hand up and your right leg forward. Alternatively, try swaying your arms from one side of your body to the other in co-ordination with your step. As you step forward with your left foot, sway both arms to your left. As you step your right foot forward, sway both arms to your right. Once you've got the hang of the arm movements, focus on making your foot movements precise. Touch the ground with your heel first – toes pointing up – then roll your foot down. Breathing is important, too. Take in two small breaths as you step forward with your left foot, and breathe out in a single exhalation as you step forward with your right foot. After 20 minutes of walking, reverse this so that you take two small inhalations as you step forward with your right foot and you exhale once as you step forward with your left foot. Do this for another 20 minutes.

Various research studies have shown that practising the standing postures of qigong can alleviate the symptoms of chronic rheumatoid arthritis. In one trial, significantly more people reported an improvement in their symptoms from practising qigong than did those from a group treated with indomethacin (a strong non-steroidal anti-inflammatory drug). Qigong can also help people with osteoarthritis of the hands, knee or hip, and with ankylosing spondylitis and non-specific muscle and joint pains.

STARTING QIGONG

You can go to classes to learn qigong or you can also learn postures and techniques from books and videos. If you can't find a dedicated qigong class, look for a tai chi class – qigong postures often form part of the class. Alternatively, a tai chi teacher may be able to offer private tuition in qigong. Try to practise qigong everyday to benefit from its therapeutic effects.

ACUPUNCTURE

Acupuncture is based on the belief that we all possess a vibrant life-energy, known as qi or chi (pronounced "chee") in China, and ki in Japan. Qi flows through the body along special channels called meridians and becomes concentrated at certain points – called acupoints – where it can enter or leave the body (see illustrations below and opposite). There are 12 main meridians and eight meridians that have a controlling function, making 20 in all. Traditionally, 365 acupoints were identified on these meridians, but many more have now been discovered and around 2,000 acupoints are illustrated on modern acupuncture charts. During acupuncture, a therapist stimulates or suppresses the flow of qi by inserting needles into your skin.

THE MERIDIANS
Meridians are energy-conducting channels that run along the length of your body. An acupuncturist inserts needles into selected acupoints that lie along these channels. This heals the body by stimulating or suppressing the flow of qi.

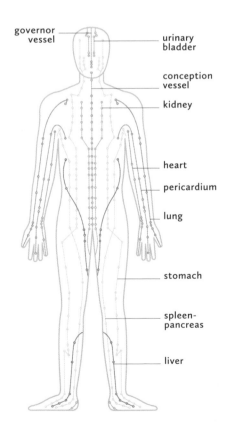

governor vessel

urinary bladder

conception vessel

kidney

heart

pericardium

lung

stomach

spleen-pancreas

liver

Acupuncture is among the most widely used complementary therapies for treating arthritis. In the West, an estimated one in two of all consultations with an acupuncturist are for arthritic conditions. Acupuncture is especially useful in the earlier stages of arthritis before degenerative changes have caused severe pain and restricted movement.

A study published in the medical journal *Rheumatology* showed that acupuncture produced a significant reduction in pain from osteoarthritis of the hip or knee after an average of eight treatments over a six-month period. Other studies show that acupuncture can relieve chronic low-back pain and neck and shoulder pain, and that it's at least as effective as treatment with non-steroidal anti-inflammatory drugs or physiotherapy.

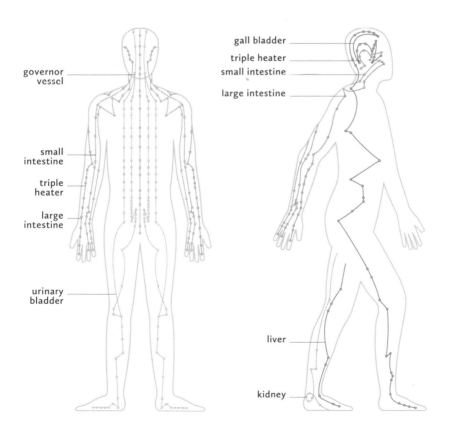

governor vessel

small intestine

triple heater

large intestine

urinary bladder

gall bladder

triple heater

small intestine

large intestine

liver

kidney

SELF-HELP ACUPRESSURE

To help reduce joint pains in your hips and lower limbs, locate an area on the base of your palm that is around a thumb's width above the wrist crease. Press either side of the midline in this area of the palm and find the point that is most tender. Press this area with the thumb of your opposite hand. Start by pressing lightly, and gradually increase the pressure as much as you can tolerate. Then release the pressure gradually and build it up again to stimulate the area. Continue pressing for about one minute, while breathing slowly and deeply. If your joint pains are worse on the left side of your body, stimulate the point on your right hand for relief, and vice versa. Do this twice a day, morning and evening.

Acupressure works on the same principles as acupuncture, but instead of inserting needles, you stimulate acupoints using firm thumb pressure or fingertip massage. You can perform acupressure on yourself (see box).

HOW ACUPUNCTURE WORKS

Acupuncture is believed to work by blocking the transmission of pain signals along nerve fibres, and by stimulating the release of endorphins, the brain's own morphine-like painkillers. It may also work by influencing the limbic system in the brain, which is involved in decisions about whether or not a sensation is perceived as painful.

VISITING AN ACUPUNCTURIST

An initial consultation usually lasts from 45 to 60 minutes, with follow-up appointments lasting around 30 minutes. The practitioner will ask about your symptoms, lifestyle, bodily functions and your emotional and physical health. He or she will examine your tongue and check various pulses in your wrists. During treatment the practitioner inserts fine, sterile, disposable needles a few millimetres into your skin at selected acupoints. Needles are usually left in place for 10 to 30 minutes and may be occasionally flicked or rotated to stimulate qi and draw or disperse energy from the point. They are sometimes stimulated with electricity (a technique known as electroacupuncture) or by burning a small cone of strong-smelling, dried Chinese herb (usually wild mugwort) near to the acupoint to warm the skin. This is known as moxibustion and is believed to stimulate weak qi in areas that are cold or painful. Acupuncturists may also stimulate acupoints using laser light from a pen-device.

For a complex, long-standing problem such as arthritis, you will benefit from having at least one treatment a week for two months. Ideally, treatment is given every other day – or even daily for acute arthritis. Most people notice an immediate benefit after just one or two treatments, while others may need up to six treatments. Information on how to find a practitioner is included at the end of this book.

REIKI

Reiki is a Japanese word meaning "universal life energy". It's a form of spiritual healing that has its roots in ancient Tibetan Buddhism and represents a simple, yet powerful way to promote emotional and physical harmony. A Reiki practitioner places their hands in a series of positions over or on your body, through which they channel and transmit the universal life energy ki. This energy is thought to help your body recover its normal state of physical and emotional wellness.

A number of studies suggest that touch therapies such as Reiki can help to reduce chronic pain and stress and improve well-being and energy levels. In one study of 82 people with osteoarthritis, pain intensity and distress were significantly reduced during the six-week period in which they received weekly Reiki sessions, compared with a similar period in which they practised progressive muscle relaxation.

VISITING A REIKI PRACTITIONER

A typical treatment session takes 60 to 90 minutes, and involves the practitioner holding his or her hands over or on your fully clothed body in 12 basic positions: four on your head, four on the front of your body, and four on your back. The practitioner holds each position for around five minutes to balance your chakras (energy centres). There are seven chakras altogether (see the illustration on page 68).

THE CHAKRAS

Life-force energy flows in to and out of the body via the chakras. When its flow is impeded, you become ill. The aim of Reiki is to restore the flow of energy in the chakras, bringing you health, and emotional and physical well-being. There are seven chakras and they lie along a line that runs from the perineum to the crown of your head. Each chakra is associated with a particular colour.

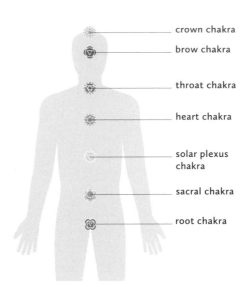

crown chakra

brow chakra

throat chakra

heart chakra

solar plexus chakra

sacral chakra

root chakra

During a healing session, your body absorbs only as much Reiki energy as it needs. You may experience the flow of energy as a mild tingling or sense of warmth or coolness. Most people experience a deep sense of relaxation, peace and well-being after treatment with Reiki. The benefits are increased by resting afterward and drinking plenty of water.

MEDITATION

Meditation is a technique that involves focusing the mind to achieve a state of peaceful relaxation and heightened awareness. This helps you to cope better with the pain of arthritis, partly because your pain perception is reduced when you're in a meditative state, and partly because meditation improves your overall mood and sense of well-being.

STARTING MEDITATION

You can go to classes to learn meditation, you can learn one-to-one from a teacher or you can simply start by yourself at home. Many yoga classes include a dedicated time for meditation. Ideally, you should meditate for 15 to 30 minutes for at least five days a week, and preferably every day.

TYPES OF MEDITATION

There are many different types of meditation – some derive from spiritual or religious backgrounds; some from secular backgrounds. These are some of the most common types in the West.

MINDFULNESS MEDITATION

This is one of the most popular forms of meditation – it encourages you to focus on the present moment. You pay close attention to everyday activities, such as preparing food, or walking, and you concentrate your awareness on the sensations, textures, colours, smells and sounds around you. Simply focusing on your breathing is also a form of mindfulness meditation. Being immersed in the moment prevents negative and stressful thoughts.

MOVING MEDITATION

This is good if you have arthritis because it involves quieting the mind through gentle movements, such as walking along a set path, or rocking or swaying to and fro. These movements are designed to keep your body engaged while your mind becomes quiet. Qigong walking is an example of moving meditation – see the box on page 63.

TRANSCENDENTAL MEDITATION

This structured form of meditation, developed by Maharishi Mahesh Yogi in the 1950s, is practised for 20 minutes twice a day. Transcendental meditation (TM) uses the silent repetition of Sanskrit mantras (short words or phrases) to still your thoughts and body so you achieve a state of restful alertness.

RELAXATION RESPONSE MEDITATION

This is a Westernized form of meditation that uses the principles of TM without the Eastern spiritual context. Instead of Sanskrit mantras, you silently chant words that are rooted in your own belief system. For example, relaxation exercises are combined with words such as "calm" or "peace".

CHAKRA MEDITATION

Chakras are worked upon in a range of complementary therapies, from yoga and Reiki, to meditation. To meditate upon the chakras sit comfortably with your eyes closed and then spend two minutes concentrating on each chakra, visualizing the colour with which it is associated. Start by focusing on the root chakra (red) at the base of your spine and imagine pulling energy up in a straight line, through the sacral chakra (orange), solar plexus chakra (yellow), heart chakra (green), throat chakra (sky blue) to the brow chakra (violet). Now focus on drawing energy up toward the crown chakra (white) at the very top of your head. Finally, imagine energy flowing out of the top of your head, like a fountain, to envelop your body in a pain-relieving, healing white light.

NUTRITIONAL APPROACHES TO TREATMENT

Research shows a definite link between the food you eat and the severity of your arthritis symptoms. Here I explain some important dietary measures that can improve your joint health. See Part Three for practical ways to implement these.

FRUIT AND VEGETABLES – EAT AT LEAST FIVE SERVINGS A DAY

Fruit and vegetables provide an array of antioxidants that reduce the rate at which cartilage breaks down, helping to slow the progression of osteoarthritis. Antioxidants can also reduce inflammation and are beneficial for people with rheumatoid arthritis, psoriatic arthritis, ankylosing spondylitis or gout. Try to eat at least five (and preferably eight or more) servings of fresh fruit and vegetables a day My full-strength program in the next section features a diet with the highest possible amount of antioxidants. See also pages 71–76.

EAT PLENTY OF OILY FISH

Oily fish are a rich source of omega-3 essential fatty acids that oil the joints and damp down inflammation. Research shows that omega-3s can reduce the need for painkillers in those with joint problems. Eat oily fish, such as salmon, sardines, herrings and mackerel, two to four times a week. You can also take an omega-3 fish-oil supplement (see page 91).

CUT DOWN ON OMEGA-6 FATS

Try to minimize your intake of vegetable oils that are rich in omega-6 essential fatty acids, such as sunflower and safflower oil – these promote inflammation. Use olive oil for cooking, and macadamia nut oil or walnut oil for salad dressings (these are rich in healthy monounsaturated fats).

DRINK PLENTY OF FLUID

Drink 2–3l (3½–5pt) of fluid a day to maintain good hydration and flow of nutrients to your joints. Choose from water, soups, tea and juices, rather than sugary soft drinks.

TRY ELIMINATION DIETS

If following the above guidelines for a healthy diet doesn't help relieve your arthritis symptoms, your joint pains may be associated with a food intolerance. If this is the case, an elimination diet may help you identify your trigger foods so that you can avoid them in future. See pages 76–77 for more details.

EAT SUPERFOODS AND TAKE SUPPLEMENTS

A number of superfoods are especially beneficial for your joint health and you should include them in your daily diet – I review them on pages 82–86. Nutritional supplements are also helpful – see pages 87–93. I also suggest specific supplement regimes for you to follow in each of the programs in Part Three.

EATING MORE ANTIOXIDANTS

Antioxidants are beneficial substances found mainly in fruit, vegetables, tea and wine. They include vitamins C and E, carotenoids, polyphenols and the mineral selenium.

WHY ANTIOXIDANTS ARE IMPORTANT

Arthritis is an inflammatory condition that is linked with the production of excess free radicals within the joints. Free radicals are unstable molecular fragments that are generated by normal metabolic reactions, exposure to pollutants, taking exercise, smoking cigarettes, drinking alcohol, bathing in UVA sunlight and taking certain drugs – including antibiotics and aspirin. Free radicals are harmful because they carry a negative electrical charge in the form of a spare electron. They try to lose this negative charge by colliding with other molecules and cell structures in an attempt to neutralize it – either by passing on their spare electron, or by stealing a positive charge. This process is called oxidation.

Each cell in your body undergoes an estimated 10,000 free-radical oxidations a day, which trigger chain reactions in which spare electrical charges are shunted from one chemical to another, damaging proteins, fats, cartilage, cell membranes and even genetic material.

Although you can't avoid generating a certain number of free radicals, you can help your joints by minimizing the amount of damage they do. Your main defence against free-radical attack is to consume as many antioxidants as possible. Antioxidants quickly mop up and neutralize the negative charges on free radicals before they can trigger a chain reaction.

RATING FOODS FOR ANTIOXIDANT POTENTIAL

To evaluate the antioxidant potential of different foods, scientists have developed a test called the Oxygen Radical Absorbance Capacity (ORAC; see page 240). This measures how well the antioxidants present in fruits and vegetables can mop up the harmful free radicals that contribute to inflammatory processes in the body, such as arthritis.

EATING MORE ANTIOXIDANTS

The amount and types of fruit and vegetables you eat have a major impact on the level of inflammation in your joints. Different foods contain different types and amounts of antioxidants of varying potency.

The average person eating a typical Western diet eats just two-and-a-half portions of fruit and vegetables a day, which provides an estimated

5,700 ORAC units. Ideally, you need to obtain at least 7,000 ORAC units a day for good health. People who eat nine servings of fruit and vegetables a day can obtain up to 20,000 ORAC units daily – this will significantly reduce the amount of free-radical damage occurring within their joints.

As well as eating plenty of servings, you also need to make informed decisions about which fruit and vegetables you eat. For example, if you eat a kiwi fruit, some watermelon, a mixed salad and some cauliflower and carrots, you would obtain fewer than 2,000 ORAC units – even though you have achieved the recommended five servings a day. On the other hand, if you eat blueberries, plums, red kidney beans, spinach and red peppers, you can rack up an astonishing 33,000 ORAC units in a single day. A number of herbs and spices have a surprisingly high ORAC score, too, even though you eat them only in small amounts. The higher your daily ORAC score, the higher your ability to neutralize free-radical damage to cells throughout your body, including your joints.

ORAC SCORES FOR HERBS AND SPICES

The following table provides you with the ORAC values for a range of herbs and spices (per gram). Adding just one gram of black pepper to a meal gives you an additional 301 ORAC units, while adding a gram of cinnamon supplies an amazing 2,675 ORAC units.

SPICE/HERB	ORAC SCORE* per gram	SPICE/HERB	ORAC SCORE* per gram
Cloves	3,144	Sage leaf	320
Cinnamon	2,675	Black peppercorns	301
Oregano	2,001	Mustard seed	292
Turmeric	1,592	Ginger powder	288
Nutmeg	1,572	Thyme	274
Cumin	768	Chilli powder	236
Parsley	743	Paprika	179
Basil leaf	676	Mint	139
Saffron	530	Garlic	54
Curry powder	485		

*ORAC score = micromol of TE (see page 240).

ORAC SCORES FOR A RANGE OF FOODS

This chart ranks a variety of foods (mostly fruit and vegetables) in terms of their ORAC score. The foods with the highest antioxidant potential per average serving are at the top.

FOOD	ORAC SCORE* per 100g	AVERAGE SERVING SIZE in grams	ORAC SCORE* per average serving
Dark chocolate	103,971	40g	41,588
Blueberries	9,260	145g	13,427
Red kidney beans	14,413	92g	13,259
Pinto beans	12,359	96g	11,864
Pomegranate	10,500	100g	10,500
Cranberries	9,456	95g	8,983
Blackberries	5,348	144g	7,701
Red lentils	9,766	75g	7,325
Prunes	8,578	85g	7,291
Globe artichoke	6,552	100g	6,552
Raspberries	4,925	123g	6,058
Strawberries	3,577	166g	5,938
Red Delicious apples	4,275	138g	5,900
Pecan nuts	17,940	28g	5,095
Cherries	3,361	145g	4,873
Plums (black)	7,339	66g	4,844
Russet potatoes (cooked)	1,555	299g	4,649
Black beans	8,040	52g	4,181
Plums (red)	6,239	66g	4,118
Gala apples	2,828	138g	3,903
Walnuts	13,541	28g	3,846
Golden Delicious apples	2,670	138g	3,685
Dates	3,895	89g	3,467
Lemons/limes	2,412	140g	3,378
Avocados	1,933	173g	3,344
Pears (green varieties)	1,911	166g	3,172
Chickpeas	4,030	75g	3,022
Pears (Red Anjou)	1,773	166g	2,943
Hazelnuts	9,645	28g	2,739
Navy beans	2,474	104g	2,573
Oranges (navel)	1,814	140g	2,540
Figs	3,383	75g	2,537
Raisins	3,037	82g	2,490

Red cabbage (cooked)	3,146	75g	2,359
Red potatoes (cooked)	1,326	173g	2,294
Pistachios	7,983	28g	2,267
Blackeye beans	4,343	52g	2,258
Green peas	4,039	50g	2,015
Red grapes	1,260	160g	2,016
Red grapefruit	1,548	123g	1,904
Beetroot	2,774	68g	1,886
Peaches	1,863	98g	1,826
Green grapes	1,118	160g	1,789
Mangoes	1,002	165g	1,653
Tangerines	1,620	84g	1,361
Pineapple	793	155g	1,229
Almonds	4,454	28g	1,265
Onions (yellow)	1,220	105g	1,281
Red leaf lettuce	1,785	68g	1,213
Sweet potatoes (cooked)	766	156g	1,195
Radishes	954	116g	1,107
Red peppers	901	119g	1,072
Spinach	2640	40g	1,056
Aubergine	2,533	41g	1,039
Bananas	879	118g	1,037
Nectarines	749	136g	1,019
Broccoli (cooked)	1,259	78g	982
Peanuts	3,166	28g	899
Carrots (raw)	1,215	61g	741
Kiwi fruit	918	76g	698
Green peppers	558	119g	664
Sweetcorn	728	77g	561
Pumpkin	483	116g	560
Tomatoes (cooked)	460	120g	552
Macadamia nuts	1,695	28g	481
Green cabbage	1,359	35g	476
Tomatoes (raw)	337	123g	415
Lemon juice	1263	30g	379
Cauliflower	647	50g	324
Watermelon	142	152g	216
Lime juice	856	30g	194
Carrots (cooked)	371	46g	171
Iceberg lettuce	451	32g	144
Cucumber (unpeeled)	115	52g	60

ELIMINATING TRIGGER FOODS

A number of foods can trigger joint pain in people with arthritis. Research shows that when avoiding foods that provoke symptoms, around 70 percent of people with all types of arthritis feel either better or much better, and report less pain, fewer painful joints, shorter duration of morning stiffness, and improved mobility and grip strength.

IDENTIFYING PROBLEM FOODS

How do you know which food or food groups – if any – you have a sensitivity to? The traditional way to find out is to follow an elimination and challenge diet (see below). However, this is time consuming and people often find it difficult to comply with the strict dietary guidelines. A number of alternative tests can help to identify problem foods; most are available only privately – for example, via a naturopath.

THE ELIMINATION AND CHALLENGE DIET

This involves following a bland, hypoallergenic diet that includes only a few, limited foods that are considered least likely to result in joint inflammation, such as:

- Grains: white rice and tapioca.
- Fruit: pears and cranberries.
- Vegetables: squash, carrots, parsnips, lettuce, lentils, and split peas.
- Meat: wild game and turkey.

After 10 days of eating this bland diet, you then start to re-introduce eliminated foods one by one, usually at three-day intervals. You keep a comprehensive food-and-symptom diary as you do this so that you can see which foods cause your joint symptoms to flare up. If you notice a link between a specific food and a worsening in your symptoms, you should avoid that food and wait until your symptoms have abated before testing another food. You can add any foods that don't trigger joint symptoms to the list of foods you can safely eat in the future.

IGG BLOOD TESTS

A blood test that measures the levels of antibodies called IgG antibodies may identify the food/s to which you are intolerant. Your blood is subjected to sophisticated testing that identifies the presence of raised levels of IgG against more than 100 food antigens.

WHITE BLOOD CELL ANALYSIS

This test assesses how your white blood cells (leukocytes) react against specific food extracts. If your white blood cells don't respond to a specific food, it's unlikely to provoke your symptoms, and you can eat it freely. However, foods that do activate your white blood cells may provoke your arthritis, and you should avoid them initially – at least for five weeks – before introducing them one by one to see which, if any, are associated with joint flare-up. Research suggests this approach can improve arthritis symptoms in as many as 83 percent of cases.

ELIMINATING NIGHTSHADE PLANTS

Some people with arthritis are particularly sensitive to foods from the nightshade (Solanaceae) family of plants. These plants produce varying amounts of chemicals known as steroidal glycoalkaloids as part of their natural defence against insects, fungi and bacteria.

Some members of the nightshade family, such as the tobacco plant, Datura (Angel's Trumpets), mandrake and Belladonna (deadly nightshade), produce toxic amounts of these alkaloids. Consuming them can trigger headache, dizziness, nausea, vomiting, diarrhea, abdominal pain, heart rhythm abnormalities, dilated pupils, muscle twitching and weakness. Other members of the nightshade family produce very small amounts of glycoalkaloids and are familiar dietary staples. Commonly eaten nightshade foods include: potatoes, tamarillo, tomatoes, physalis, aubergine, sweet peppers, chilli peppers, paprika, cayenne and all other types of pepper, except black pepper, which belongs to a different family (Piperaceae). Unlike many other plant toxins, glycoalkaloids are not broken down or detoxified by cooking, baking, or frying, which does, in fact, concentrate them.

YOUR TRIGGER FOODS

The foods most commonly found to worsen arthritis symptoms are: wheat, corn, rye, sugar, caffeine, yeast, malt, dairy products, oranges, grapefruit, lemons and tomatoes. The types of meats most likely to provoke symptoms are bacon, pork, beef and lamb. However, some of these foods are also arthritis superfoods and can actually help to improve joint health. Food intolerances are highly specific to the individual – culprit foods vary from one person to another. It's therefore important to keep a food-and-symptom diary to help pinpoint foods that provoke your symptoms. This is not always an easy task, as symptoms can sometimes worsen up to 36 hours after eating a trigger food.

Why some people seem to experience a flare-up in joint symptoms as a result of eating nightshade plants is not fully understood, but it's possible that glycoalkaloids may trigger joint inflammation through an immune system mechanism or by altering calcium metabolism in bone. Another possible explanation relates to the recent finding that glycoalkaloids have an adverse effect on intestinal permeability to increase gut leakiness. This may increase the presence of other food allergens in the circulation, which may provoke the immune system into mounting a response. This mechanism has also been suggested as a cause or aggravator of inflammatory bowel disorders such as Crohn's disease and ulcerative colitis – autoimmune conditions that are often accompanied by an inflammatory type of arthritis.

If you want to try eliminating nightshade foods from your diet, be prepared to wait for an improvement in your joint symptoms. It takes more than 24 hours for ingested glycoalkaloids to be cleared from your body, and if you eat foods containing them every day, they can accumulate in your body. You will usually notice the beneficial effects of eliminating nightshade foods within two to three weeks.

Research dating back to 1979 suggests that eliminating nightshade foods from the diet can improve arthritis symptoms in more than 70 percent of people with osteoarthritis, rheumatoid arthritis, and other joint problems. I explain how to eliminate nightshade foods in the moderate program (see pages 152–191).

ELIMINATING MEAT

Studies have shown a link between the amount of meat fat, meat and offal consumed in a country and the number of people with an inflammatory type of arthritis. It has also been suggested that eating a vegan or lactovegetarian diet can reduce the number of affected joints and shorten the duration of morning stiffness in people with rheumatoid arthritis.

Inflammatory arthritis is associated with intestinal inflammation, increased gut permeability and raised levels of antibodies directed against gut bacteria and food antigens. Researchers have found similarities in the amino acid make-up of a cow protein (bovine albumin) and human collagen (present in joint cartilage). It's possible that if the body mounts an immune response to eating beef, the antibodies that are intended to attack the cow protein may attack human joints, too.

Switching to a lactovegetarian or vegan diet can also help joint symptoms by normalizing the pattern of bacteria present in the gut and increasing the number of probiotic bacteria. The pattern of bacteria found in the bowel of people with early rheumatoid arthritis is significantly different from that in healthy people without rheumatoid arthritis. An abnormal pattern of bowel bacteria may result in the production of chemicals that increase joint inflammation.

Another advantage of eating a vegetarian diet is that you're likely to have an increased intake of anti-inflammatory antioxidants, including alphacarotene, betacarotene, lycopene, lutein, vitamin C and vitamin E.

VEGAN DIETS

As a vegan diet is associated with reduced intakes of vitamins B12 and D, people switching to a vegan diet should consider taking a vitamin-B12 supplement and, if sun exposure is limited, a vitamin-D supplement, too.

ELIMINATING "ACID" FOODS

It's possible, for a reason that isn't yet understood, that foods classified as "acid" may increase joint inflammation. In fact, the advice given by some naturopaths to people with arthritis is to eat a diet that consists of 60 to 80 percent alkaline foods and 20 to 40 percent acid foods.

There's a lot of confusion around the terms "acid" and "alkaline". They refer to the effects certain foods have on the pH of your urine – not whether the food itself is acidic or alkaline in quality, and not the effect it has on the acidity of your digestive system or even your blood. This is because your body works hard to keep the fluids bathing your cells within a very tight pH range of 7.35–7.45, which is slightly alkaline. If your blood pH falls even slightly outside of this range, you will become quite ill. This is because your metabolism relies on a constant, low level of alkalinity in order to work properly.

When food is broken down, its various building blocks – proteins, carbohydrates and fats – are metabolized to result in either the production or the consumption of protons. These are positively charged hydrogen ions (H+), the concentration of which determines the pH of a fluid. If the metabolism of a food results in the production of excess protons, it's classified as an acid food ("acid-forming" is a more accurate description). If the metabolism of a food uses up more protons than it produces, then it's classified as an alkaline (or alkaline-forming) food.

ACID- AND ALKALINE-FORMING FOODS

ACID-FORMING

Vegetables with a high protein or sulphur content: grains (barley, oats, quinoa, rice, wheat); pulses (for example, black beans, chickpeas, kidney beans, lentils and soybeans), most nuts (pecans, cashews, peanuts, pistachios and walnuts)
Some fruits: blueberries, cranberries, plums, prunes
Dairy products: cheese, milk, ice-cream, yogurt
Animal proteins: eggs, poultry, meat, seafood
Alcohol: beer, wine

ALKALINE-FORMING

Mildly alkaline: low-sugar fruit, such as sour cherries; berries; grapefruit; lemons; limes; peppers
Strongly alkaline: graeen leafy vegetables, such as kale, broccoli and spinach; avocado; tomato

So, although some foods such as oranges, lemons, limes and tomatoes are acid to taste, the way their building blocks are metabolized in your body means they are classified as alkaline foods. In fact, fruit is your main dietary source of alkali. In contrast, protein-rich foods, such as meat and dairy products, are acid-forming. As amino acids – the building blocks of protein – are broken down, excess protons are produced. Your body gets rid of the acidity in the form of acidic carbon dioxide gas exhaled via your lungs, but some excess acid is also voided in your urine.

Not everyone is sensitive to acid-forming foods. If you can tolerate aspirin without experiencing a worsening in joint symptoms, then you're unlikely to have a problem with acid-forming foods. I don't recommend that you limit your intake of acid-forming foods until you have tried other therapeutic dietary approaches (see Part Three) first. If you've done this and you still haven't got adequate symptom relief, try limiting acid-forming foods under the supervision of a qualified medical nutritionist. Many acid-forming foods are also important sources of protein, vitamins, minerals and antioxidants – a medical nutritionist will tell you how to how best to replace these in your diet.

ELIMINATING PURINE-RICH FOODS

Gout is a type of inflammatory arthritis that's caused by high levels of uric acid in joints and tissues. Uric acid comes from the breakdown of substances called purines in the body. Most of the uric acid we produce comes from the breakdown of purines that are released when the genetic material (DNA) of worn-out cells is recycled. However, some foods also contain purines and changing your diet to eliminate purines can lower uric acid levels in your body by up to 20 percent. The following foods are rich in purines and you should avoid them if you have gout: shellfish and oily fish; offal, meat and game; yeast extract; asparagus; and spinach. I also suggest that you avoid alcohol – it both increases uric-acid production and reduces its excretion. Cut out beer, especially, which is very rich in purines.

SUPERFOODS FOR ARTHRITIS

The food and drinks in this chart have a natural anti–inflammatory action that's particularly beneficial for people with arthritis. Try to incorporate at least five of these superfoods into your diet every day. However, avoid foods that trigger an idiosyncratic reaction and worsen your arthritis.

SUPERFOOD	BENEFITS	HOW TO USE IT
Apples Contain anti-inflammatory antioxidants and bone-friendly boron and magnesium. Red Delicious apples contain the most antioxidants in their skin and flesh.	Eating 100g/3½oz apple provides the same antioxidant benefits as 1,500mg vitamin C. Wash but don't peel your apples – the antioxidants are five times more concentrated in the skin than the flesh.	Eat as a daily snack. Grate (mix with lemon juice to prevent browning) and add to salads and coleslaw. Eat dried apple rings and apple crisps. Cloudy apple juice has more antioxidants than clear.
Avocado Contains antioxidant monounsaturated oils, essential fatty acids, beta-sitosterol and vitamin E.	Avocado can suppress joint inflammation by reducing production of inflammatory substances. It promotes cartilage repair in osteoarthritis by stimulating the activity of bone-building cells and cartilage cells.	Use an avocado slicer to easily remove flesh from the skin. Eat as a starter and add to salads. Mash to make dips (for example, guacamole) or simply spread onto oatcakes.
Brazil nuts The richest dietary source of selenium – a single Brazil nut contains around 50mcg. Selenium improves the quality of cartilage proteins. Also a good source of magnesium and sulphur.	People with the highest dietary intake of selenium are least likely to develop osteoarthritis. Each increase of 0.1 parts per million of selenium in your toenail clippings (a good indicator of selenium status) lowers your risk of knee osteoarthritis by 20 percent.	Eat as a snack. Scatter over cereal, yogurts and salads. Brazil nut butter is a delicious spread. Buy little and often for maximum freshness.

Chilli peppers Contain substances called capsaicin and dihydrocapsaicin.

Capsaicin and dihydrocapsaicin block transmission of pain messages. They also trigger the release of endorphins – the brain's own morphine-like painkillers. Capsaicin is used in clinical trials as a long-acting analgesic to treat post-surgical and osteoarthritis pain – a single injection acts for several months.

Add chilli pepper to curries, soups and stews. Use sweet chilli jelly as a conserve with meats and cheeses.

Curry powder spices For example, anise, chilli, cloves, cumin, fennel, ginger, mustard and turmeric.

Curry spices have an anti-inflammatory, painkilling action. Mustard reduces inflammation in a similar way to aspirin. Turmeric and ginger contain curcumin, which may reduce cartilage destruction in osteoarthritis, and prevent the onset of rheumatoid arthritis.

Increase your consumption of spiced Indian and Middle-Eastern foods.

Dark green leafy vegetables For example, broccoli, spinach, spring greens, dark green cabbage and parsley. These vegetables supply antioxidant carotenoids, vitamin C, calcium and magnesium.

A high antioxidant diet is good for arthritis (see pages 71–73). Sixty-one percent of the bone-friendly calcium found in broccoli is absorbed from the gut, compared with only 32 percent of calcium in milk.

Steam greens lightly to accompany meals. Use raw baby spinach leaves in salads. Add leaves to the mix when juicing fruit and vegetables.

Dark blue-red pigmented fruits For example, cherries, grapes, blueberries, bilberries, dark raspberries and elderberries. These contain antioxidant anthocyanins.

Anthocyanins lower levels of inflammatory chemicals in the body. Eating 250g/9oz black cherries daily can lower uric acid levels enough to prevent gout. Drinking a glass of red grape juice has an antioxidant action that lasts for two hours.

Eat fresh or frozen. Add to yogurt, muesli, fromage frais, fruit salads or any other dessert. Purée to make a coulis. Juice berries and dilute with apple juice for a refreshing, antioxidant-rich drink.

Garlic Contains beneficial substances such as allicin.

A Russian study has shown that people with rheumatoid arthritis can alleviate symptoms by increasing the amount of garlic they eat.

Add to all savoury dishes just before the end of cooking.

Grapefruit Contains vitamin C and antioxidant bioflavonoids. Red grapefruit has a higher antioxidant content than yellow grapefruit.

Grapefruit helps to reduce inflammation, strengthen cartilage and block prostaglandins (substances involved in pain). It increases the anti-inflammatory effect of some painkillers. Eating grapefruit regularly improves symptoms in some people with rheumatoid and other forms of inflammatory arthritis.

Eat as a starter; add to fruit salads; drink the freshly-squeezed juice. Check for drug interactions by asking the pharmacist who dispenses your usual prescriptions.

Macadamias The richest food source of monounsaturated fatty acids and an excellent source of vitamin E and selenium.

The antioxidant action reduces inflammation in arthritis. Macadamia nuts are being used in a trial to reduce the risk of rheumatoid arthritis.

Eat a handful as a snack; scatter over cereal, yogurts and salads. Macadamia nut butter is a delicious spread.

Milk A good source of calcium and B-vitamins.

People who drink milk daily are significantly less likely to have clinical or x-ray evidence of knee osteoarthritis than those with a lower level of consumption (after taking other dietary factors into account).

Pour over cereals for breakfast; add to drinks such as tea; and use to make smoothies, shakes and milk puddings.

Mushrooms Medicinal mushrooms such as *Tricholoma giganteum*, reishi (*Ganoderma lucidum*), maitake (*Grifola frondosa*), and *Phellinus linteus* contain immune-modulating substances.

Medicinal mushrooms can inhibit production of inflammatory substances in experimental models of arthritis.

Slice into salads; make into soup; sauté in olive oil with garlic; bake stuffed with mashed butternut squash and parsley. Take reishi or maitake supplements.

Oily fish A rich source of anti-inflammatory omega-3 fatty acids (EPA and DHA).

A large analysis of 17 studies assessing the pain-relieving effects of omega-3 fatty acids in rheumatoid and other autoimmune forms of arthritis showed they significantly reduce joint pain and intensity, the duration of morning stiffness, the number of painful joints, and the need to take NSAIDs – all within three to four months.

Eat fish that's as fresh as possible, and preferably raw (for example, sushi and sashimi), steamed, grilled or baked until just set. Eat two to four portions of oily fish a week – girls and women who may get pregnant in the future should limit their intake to two portions a week to reduce their exposure to mercury.

Olive oil A rich source of monounsaturated fats, and antioxidant, anti-inflammatory substances.

Increased olive oil consumption is associated with a reduced risk of rheumatoid arthritis and cardiovascular disease. Olive oil may protect against the development of osteoarthritis.

Use plain olive oil for cooking. Use extra virgin olive oil (made from the first pressing of the olives) in salad dressings and for drizzling on food (it has the highest antioxidant content, but smokes at high heat).

Onions A rich source of quercetin – an antioxidant bioflavonoid that suppresses the production of inflammatory substances. Red onions are particularly high in antioxidants.

Quercetin binds to cartilage and strengthens its structure. As an antioxidant it mops up free radicals within joints and reduces the release of protein-degrading enzymes.

Make French onion soup. Serve onion sauces and onion marmalade with meat dishes. Slice raw red onions into salads.

Pomegranate A rich source of antioxidant polyphenols, anthocyanins, vitamins C and E and carotenoids. Its antioxidant potential is two or three times higher than that of red wine and green tea.

Ellagic acid in pomegranate juice reduces inflammation by blocking activation of inflammatory substances that play a key role in cartilage degradation in osteoarthritis.

Buy fresh pomegranate juice drinks or make your own. Add pomegranate seeds to salads and desserts.

Red wine A rich source of antioxidant polyphenols such as resveratrol.

Resveratrol blocks the release of inflammatory substances, which helps to reduce joint inflammation.

Drink one or two glasses, once or twice a week (as long as wine doesn't worsen your arthritis symptoms).

Soybeans These contain antioxidant isoflavones that have a beneficial oestrogen-like action to strengthen bones.

Soy suppresses joint inflammation and pain. It blocks production of inflammatory substances in joints and promotes the repair of cartilage in osteoarthritis by stimulating the activity of osteoblasts (bone-building cells) and chondrocytes (cartilage cells).

Use soybeans in soups, stews and stir fries. Use tofu and soy sauce in cooking. Add soybean protein powder to shakes.

Teas White, green, oolong and black teas contain high levels of antioxidant catechins, such as epigallocatechin-3-gallate (EGCG).

EGCG inhibits the expression of inflammatory mediators in arthritic joints and helps to protect cartilage degradation in osteoarthritis.

Drink green, black or white tea regularly, three to five times a day. Use left-over cold tea to soak dried fruit. Use green or white tea as a basis for sauces, soups or stews or to make ice cream.

Walnuts A rich source of omega-3 fatty acids.

Omega-3 fatty acids have an anti-inflammatory action. Some research shows that eating walnuts daily can help alleviate the symptoms of rheumatoid arthritis.

Add chopped walnuts to cereals, salads, vegetarian dishes and desserts. Use walnut butter as a spread.

Yellow or orange fruit and vegetables For example, carrots, sweet potatoes, guava, mango and pumpkin – these are all rich sources of vitamin C and antioxidant carotenoids.

Fruit and vegetables with a high antioxidant content can reduce pain and inflammation in all types of arthritis.

Eat fresh in fruit salads or on its own for dessert. Purée to make fruit coulis, shakes and smoothies. Dried mango makes a deliciously healthy sweet snack (avoid those preserved with sulfites).

Yogurt (live) Contains probiotic bacteria.

Probiotic bacteria help to reduce the severity of joint inflammation. They also reduce abnormal intestinal bacterial balance (dysbiosis) associated with "leakiness" of the gut wall and food intolerance.

Eat low-fat bio yogurt with breakfast cereals, and with chopped fruit in desserts. Drink probiotic yogurt drinks.

SUPPLEMENTS FOR ARTHRITIS

These are the supplements that I believe are of most benefit to your joint health, easing pain and stiffness and improving mobility. They also help to alleviate the symptoms of both osteoarthritis and autoimmune arthritis. Whereas prescribed drugs such as NSAIDs (see pages 28–29) can only damp down inflammation and pain, some supplements, such as glucosamine and chondroitin, have the potential to halt the degenerative changes of osteoarthritis.

Each supplement tends to be effective for two out of three people with joint pain, so choose a supplement and try it for a couple of months until you find one that works for you. Most joint health supplements can be taken together for additional, synergistic benefits. As well as being as effective as some prescribed analgesics, supplements are less likely to cause adverse side effects.

SUPPLEMENT	RESEARCH FINDINGS	DOSE AND COMMENTS
Vitamin B5 (pantothenic acid) This is vital for many energy-producing reactions in the body. It also stimulates cell growth in healing tissues. Vitamin B5 is rapidly depleted during times of stress.	Lack of vitamin B5 causes defects in cartilage formation. Blood levels of B5 are lower than normal in people with rheumatoid arthritis. When people with rheumatoid arthritis were given B5 injections, symptoms improved in most cases but recurred when supplementation was discontinued. Oral supplements of calcium pantothenate can reduce the duration of morning stiffness, degree of disability and severity of pain in rheumatoid arthritis.	An intake of 4–7mg is believed to be adequate. Nutritional therapists may prescribe higher doses of 50–200mg daily.

Vitamin B6 Needed to lower levels of homocysteine – a harmful, inflammatory amino acid that can cause hardening and furring up of the arteries (atherosclerosis).

People with rheumatoid arthritis have low B6 levels, raised homocysteine levels and an increased risk of heart disease. Vitamin B6 may help alleviate carpal tunnel syndrome (CTS), which can affect people with osteoarthritis of the wrist. It can also reduce hand pain in osteoarthritis.

An intake of 2mg daily is believed to be adequate. Nutritional therapists may prescribe higher doses of 10–200mg daily.

Folate (Vitamin B9) Needed to lower homocysteine levels.

Can reduce hand pain in osteoarthritis by reducing systemic inflammation.

Nutritional therapists recommend 400–1000 mcg daily. Folic acid – the synthetic form of folate – is more easily absorbed and used in the body than the naturally occurring folate. Take with vitamin B12 to avoid masking B12 deficiency.

Vitamin B12 Needed to lower homocysteine levels.

Levels of vitamin B12 tend to be low in people with rheumatoid arthritis, psoriatic arthropathy and lupus, and this contributes to a high incidence of anemia.

The usual recommended intake is 1mcg daily. Nutritional therapists recommend up to 1000mcg daily.

Vitamin C (ascorbic acid) This is a powerful antioxidant. It's needed for the production of collagen in ligaments and cartilage.

Lack of vitamin C may contribute to cartilage ageing. Vitamin C supplements can reduce osteoarthritic hip and knee pain. In a study of 640 men and women, those with moderate to high intakes of vitamin C (two or more times the recommended daily amount) were three times less likely to develop knee pain or see their knee osteoarthritis progress than those with a lower intake of vitamin C (up to about twice the recommended daily amount).

The usual recommended intake is 60–120mg daily. Nutritional therapists recommend up to 1–3g daily. Vitamin C supplements may cause indigestion – to overcome this, use ester-C, a non-acidic form that is more readily absorbed and used by the body.

Vitamin D This is essential for the absorption of dietary calcium and phosphate in the small intestine, and for the deposition of calcium and phosphate in bone, and for bone modelling. It can be synthesized in the body by the action of sunlight (UVB rays) on the skin.

Cartilage and bone is sensitive to lack of vitamin D. In people with low vitamin D, hip osteoarthritis is more likely. Osteoarthritis can progress three to four times more rapidly in some people with vitamin D deficiency. Vitamin D supplements can relieve joint pain in some people with osteoarthritis. People low in vitamin D are also 33 percent more likely to develop rheumatoid arthritis.

The usual recommended intake is 5–10mcg. Up to 25mcg daily isn't thought to be harmful.

Vitamin E This is a powerful antioxidant, which blocks the action of inflammatory prostaglandins to relieve pain, and also helps to stabilize joint cartilage.

People with the highest intake of vitamin E are half as likely to develop knee osteoarthritis as those with the lowest intakes. Research shows that vitamin E is twice as effective as a placebo or simple analgesics in reducing pain levels in some people with osteoarthritis. Low vitamin E levels appear to increase the risk of developing rheumatoid arthritis.

The usual recommended intake is 10mg daily. Nutritional therapists may prescribe higher doses of up to 727mg (800IU) daily. Take together with vitamin C, which is needed to regenerate vitamin E.

Boron A trace mineral that plays a role in bone calcium metabolism by boosting production of the active form of vitamin D.

Bone boron levels are lower than normal in people with arthritis. In areas where boron intakes are low (less than or equal to 1mg daily), the incidence of arthritis ranges from 20–70 percent, but where boron intakes are good (3–10mg daily), the incidence of arthritis is 10 percent or less. Boron appears to protect against both osteoarthritis and rheumatoid arthritis, but the mechanism remains unknown.

A daily intake of 3mg is suggested as optimum for bone health. Nutritional therapists may prescribe higher doses of 3–9mg per day as part of a multivitamin and mineral supplement.

Calcium A mineral that is vital for the maintenance of strong, healthy bones.

People with arthritis have reduced mobility and are at risk of future osteoporosis, especially if their intake of calcium is low and/or they take corticosteroids. Calcium supplements can improve bone strength in people with all types of arthritis.

Intakes of 800–1000mg are needed for optimal bone health. Nutritional therapists may prescribe doses of 300–1,500mg. High doses should usually be taken together with other minerals such as zinc, iron and magnesium. Calcium tablets are best taken with meals. People who tend to suffer from kidney stones should take calcium supplements together with essential fatty acids (ask your doctor about this).

Magnesium A mineral that is important for the action of virtually all body enzymes, and for maintaining the integrity of cells.

People with rheumatoid arthritis tend to have low magnesium levels and reduced activity of this enzyme. Low levels of magnesium contribute to fatigue.

300mg daily. Make sure you maintain a good calcium intake when you take magnesium supplements.

Selenium A trace element needed to make powerful antioxidant enzymes (glutathione peroxidases) that reduce inflammation in the body. Selenium also increases the effectiveness of vitamin E.

Lack of selenium is associated with greater severity of osteoarthritis and rheumatoid arthritis.

Intakes of around 75mcg are believed to be adequate. Nutritional therapists may recommend doses of 50–200mcg. Selenium that's organically bound to yeast is more readily absorbed and usable than selenium salts.

Zinc An essential trace element needed for the action of over a hundred different enzymes. It helps to regulate gene activation and the synthesis of specific proteins.

People with rheumatoid arthritis tend to have a reduced ability to absorb zinc, and a lower than normal zinc level. Supplements supplying zinc sulphate appear to have a beneficial action in psoriatic arthropathy, and to reduce the need for painkillers.

15mg daily.

Evening primrose oil A source of an anti-

Research shows that taking evening primrose oil for

Take 500mg to 3g daily. This is equivalent to 40mg

inflammatory omega-6 essential fatty acid called gammalinolenic acid (GLA).

three months may enable people with rheumatoid arthritis to reduce their NSAID dose. Evening primrose oil can also reduce fatigue in people with rheumatoid arthritis.

and 240mg GLA. Do not take evening primrose oil if you have a rare disorder known as temporal lobe epilepsy.

Omega-3 fish oils A rich source of omega-3 fatty acids, EPA and DHA (eicosapentaenoic acid and docosahexaenoic acid).

EPA and DHA damp down inflammation and can reduce the long-term need for painkillers in people with joint pain. They may also reduce the risk of coronary heart disease in people with rheumatoid arthritis.

Take 500mg to 4g daily. For severe inflammatory disease, nutritional therapists may recommend up to 6g daily. Fish oils can cause belching and mild nausea. Seek medical advice before taking fish-oil supplements if you have a blood-clotting disorder or are taking a blood-thinning drug such as aspirin or warfarin (fish oils may increase the tendency to bleed). If you have diabetes, monitor your glucose levels carefully when taking fish-oil supplements.

Cod liver oil (CLO) Contains omega-3 essential fatty acids and vitamins A and D.

Cod liver oil can reduce musculoskeletal pain. It may also reduce incidence of gastrointestinal side effects produced by NSAIDs.

Take "extra high strength" or "concentrated" supplements. Do not take cod liver oil supplements during pregnancy.

Green-lipped mussel extracts Contain an omega-3 fatty acid (eicosatetraenoic acid) that inhibits the production of a group of inflammatory substances in the body.

A 2003 study found these extracts significantly improved the signs and symptoms of osteoarthritis by 53 percent within one month, and 80 percent within two months. A clinical trial involving 30 people with rheumatoid arthritis and 30 with osteoarthritis found significant benefit for 23 with the rheumatoid condition and 21 with osteoarthritis.

Take 200–1200mg daily. Supplements are available in powdered or oil form.

Glucosamine A natural substance needed for the repair of cartilage, but one that's often in short supply. It's used to both treat and prevent osteoarthritis.

Glucosamine sulphate supplements can improve osteoarthritis symptoms by as much as 73 percent and are at least as effective as paracetamol in reducing pain. A trial published in *The Lancet* (2001) showed that taking 1500mg glucosamine daily produced significant improvements in pain and disability in people with osteoarthritis of the knee, with no significant loss of joint space over the three-year trial period. And a systematic review of 20 trials found, in people with osteoarthritis, glucosamine was more effective at relieving pain than a placebo – with a 28 percent improvement in pain and a 21 percent improvement in joint function.

Take 1000–2000mg daily. Glucosamine is often combined with other ingredients such as chondroitin, selenium or MSM to increase its effectiveness.

Chondroitin sulphate This attracts water into joints, which acts as a shock absorber, as well as a nutrient transport system. It inhibits enzymes that break down cartilage, while stimulating those involved in the production of structural substances. It is used to treat osteoarthritis.

Research shows that taking chondroitin significantly improves pain and joint function in people with osteoarthritis of the knee within three months. In people taking a placebo, joint space width decreased, while in those taking chondroitin, there was no deterioration in joint space.

Take 800–1600mg daily. Chondroitin is often combined with glucosamine – the two supplements have a naturally synergistic action.

MSM (methyl-sulphonyl-methane) A sulphur compound that has an anti-inflammatory action. It reduces the formation of free radicals by white blood cells.

MSM can reduce pain in people with osteoarthritis by 82 percent within six weeks, compared with an average improvement of 18 percent in those taking a placebo. The combination of 500mg glucosamine plus 500mg MSM three times a

Take 1–2g daily, in divided doses. MSM is often taken together with glucosamine.

day can significantly improve joint function and reduce pain and swelling more than either supplement on its own. The combination also produces a more rapid improvement in symptoms.

Garlic Provides allicin (diallyl thiosulphinate), which is a powerful antioxidant and a source of sulphur. It has an anti-inflammatory action related to that of MSM.

A Russian study has shown that 86 percent of people with rheumatoid arthritis who took a garlic supplement experienced a reduction in arthritis symptoms within four to six weeks, with no side effects.

Take 600–900mg daily. Select tablets standardized to provide 1000–1500mcg allicin. Choose products with an enteric coating – this reduces odour and protects active ingredients from degradation in the stomach.

Collagen hydrolysates These are essentially gelatin obtained from the carcasses of chickens, pigs, sheep or cows. They provide building blocks such as chondroitin sulphate for joint repair and may reduce pain in those with severe symptoms of arthritis.

Collagen hydrolysates may help promote joint cartilage renewal. In a six-month study of 100 older people, those taking collagen hydrolysates showed significant improvement in joint mobility compared with those taking a placebo.

Take 300mg to 1g daily.

CMO (cis-9-cetyl myristoleate) This is a waxy oil containing cetylated fatty acids. It acts as a joint lubricant and has an anti-inflammatory action. It's used to treat all types of arthritis.

CMO helps to lubricate joints and can reduce pain either when taken in oral form, or when rubbed on to a joint as a cream. Research has shown that 68 days of taking oral CMO can bring about a significant increase in the range of knee movement in people with osteoarthritis, improving flexion by 10 degrees.

Take 300–600mg daily. You can take CMO with an enzyme (lipase), to aid its digestion. Tobacco, alcohol and caffeine use are reported to reduce the effectiveness of CMO.

LIFESTYLE APPROACHES TO TREATMENT

Changing aspects of your lifestyle can bring about dramatic improvements in the way you feel. For example, something as basic as losing weight can relieve pressure on your joints and go a long way to easing pain and stiffness. Here are some of the most important adjustments you can make to your lifestyle to relieve joint symptoms and maximize joint health.

QUIT SMOKING

Smoking is a risk factor for developing rheumatoid arthritis, and it increases disease activity and severity once you have rheumatoid arthritis. It also hastens the hardening and furring up of your arteries and has a more dangerous effect on artery walls in people with rheumatoid arthritis than in the general population. For people with osteoarthritis of the knee, smoking is associated with increased cartilage loss and pain. Some studies also suggest that smoking is associated with low-back pain. These effects may be related to blood-vessel constriction and a reduced supply of oxygen and nutrients to joints and intervertebral discs.

DRINK IN MODERATION

If you drink too much alcohol, you're at an increased risk of developing rheumatoid arthritis. Alcohol is toxic to muscle cells and may also increase the risk of tendon rupture in people with inflammatory disease. Limiting your alcohol intake is also an easy way to cut back on calories. Aim to drink no more than two or three units of alcohol a day.

TIPS TO HELP YOU QUIT SMOKING
- Find support – stopping smoking is much easier when you do it with a friend.
- Suck on artificial cigarettes or chew carrot sticks to help overcome cravings.
- Consider using nicotine replacement products or nicotine-trapping drops (available from pharmacies) that you add to cigarette filters.
- Keep your hands busy – draw, knit, paint, or play with worry beads.

FIND WAYS TO DEAL WITH STRESS

Prolonged stress lowers your pain threshold and increases your perception of joint pain. Stress can also increase disease activity in rheumatoid arthritis. Try to avoid stressful situations through forward planning and learn to say "no" when unreasonable demands are made on you. If you start to feel stressed, stop what you are doing, take a deep breath, and inwardly say "calm" to yourself. Try listening to calming music to help you unwind; and place a few drops of a flower essence such as Rescue Remedy under your tongue. Many of the complementary therapies in Part Two can reduce the effects of stress – try aromatherapy, yoga, qigong, massage, reflexology, acupressure and meditation.

CHOOSE A GOOD MATTRESS

Many people with arthritis sleep on a mattress that is too hard or too soft, and this can make joint pain worse. Scientists have now developed the perfect sleeping surface – a visco-elastic polymer that is heat and pressure sensitive and naturally moulds to your body. This "memory foam" gives firm support as your body sinks into the material, supporting the curves of your back, reducing the load on pressure points and helping muscles and ligaments recover during sleep. Reduction of strain on your pressure points also reduces the number of times you turn during sleep from 50 to 80 times a night to around 20. This alleviates restlessness and pain, which in turn reduces the need for sleeping tablets and painkillers.

CHOOSE SHOES THAT REDUCE JOINT STRESS

Exercise and weight loss can improve pain from knee arthritis, but until recently little attention was paid to the design of shoes. Masai Barefoot Technology (MBT) make shoes with a reverse heel that mimics walking on unstable ground. This forces you to walk more naturally in an upright manner. MBT shoes dynamically alter weight loading so pressure is distributed evenly through your foot from the moment your heel strikes the ground to the moment your toes lift off. Research shows that wearing

MBT shoes can reduce stress on knee and hip joints by around 20 percent, and increase muscle activity in your lower limbs and thigh muscles by a similar amount. Many osteopaths, chiropractors, physiotherapists and orthopedic surgeons recommend MBT shoes to treat lower back pain and arthritis – the shoes are available in more than 20 countries and are classed as medical devices in the EU. Trials show that they can improve pain, stiffness and physical functioning by at least 10 percent, with benefits occurring within the first three to six weeks.

USE A WALKING AID

Using a walking stick improves balance and more than halves the load on a damaged leg joint. If you have pain or weakness on one side, hold the stick in the opposite hand. When walking, start by putting all your weight on your stronger leg. Now step forward with your affected leg and the walking stick at the same time. This allows you to support your weight on a combination of your affected leg and the stick, so you can now step forward using your stronger leg.

To walk upstairs, put your stronger leg on the first step, then bring your affected leg and the walking stick onto the same step. Repeat these actions, so you go up the steps one by one. To walk downstairs, start by lowering your bad leg and the walking stick on to the top step. Next, bring your better leg down on to that same step and continue going down one step at a time. Always keep your free hand on the railing.

If you're using a walking stick to help you balance, then use whichever hand makes you feel most comfortable and stable. Place the stick firmly on the ground and step forward only once you feel secure.

USE OTHER LIFESTYLE AIDS

A variety of assistive devices can make life more comfortable. For example, wedge a lumbar support between your seat and your lower back to make sitting easier. And wear a joint support around affected joints to keep them warm and stable. When travelling, support your head on a U-shaped travel pillow to mimimize jolts and to relieve neck pain; and use soft pillows on armrests.

TAKING REGULAR EXERCISE

Whatever form of arthritis you have, gentle exercise helps to maintain your joint mobility and function and provides reductions in pain and disability. Yet many people with arthritis don't exercise because they fear it will make their joints worse.

THE BENEFITS OF EXERCISE
Researchers have found that particular forms of exercise may have a positive effect on joint health in people with osteoarthritis and rheumatoid arthritis.

OSTEOARTHRITIS
Exercise can postpone the onset of osteoarthritis or slow its progress if you already have it. When researchers from Stanford University, California, compared 538 members of a running club with 423 people who never exercised, they found that running offers up to 12 years protection against the onset of osteoarthritis. Those who ran between 10 and 32km (six and 20 miles) a week gained the most benefit. All participants were aged around 58 and were assessed regularly for pain and disability, as well as having the progression of osteoarthritis checked using x-rays. Twenty percent of those who took no exercise had pain and disability compared with only five percent of the runners, with women being at greatest risk of disability. Other studies suggest that strength training may slow knee arthritis, and lower body exercises can reduce the rate of space narrowing in the knee joint.

Some researchers believe that weight-bearing exercise, such as running, is helpful because it encourages the production of synovial fluid which helps to lubricate the joints. However, excessive running can put joints under strain. Also, any sport that twists the joints, such as football or rugby, can cause tearing and injury which is a risk factor for developing osteoarthritis, especially in the knee.

A study called the Fitness, Arthritis and Seniors Trial (FAST) involved 435 people with knee osteoarthritis, aged 60 or over – they were randomly assigned to an 18-month health-education program, a weight-training program or an aerobic-exercise program. The participants who did aerobic exercise showed the biggest improvements in walking speed and the biggest reductions in pain and disability. Another study involving 100 people over the age of 60 who had knee arthritis showed that exercise – whether walking or weight training – improved stability and reduced the tendency to sway while standing. And for people with osteoarthritis of the hands, home exercises can help to protect the joints and can increase grip strength by 25 percent.

RHEUMATOID ARTHRITIS

If you're struggling to cope with both the pain and fatigue of rheumatoid arthritis, aerobic exercise may seem impossible. In the past people with rheumatoid arthritis were advised to do only non-weight-bearing, isometric exercises because of concerns that more intensive exercise might worsen pain and damage joints. However, we now know that aerobic exercise is the most helpful form of exercise. It not only improves your muscle strength and joint mobility, it also increases your cardiorespiratory fitness.

People with rheumatoid arthritis who exercise more than three times a week for at least 20 minutes have significantly less fatigue and disability after six months when compared with non-exercisers. And these benefits occur without any increase in pain and without any apparent worsening of disease activity or arthritis progression. Long-term, high-intensity, weight-bearing exercises may even have a protective effect on certain joints, such as those in the feet, and can slow down the loss of bone-mineral density at the hip.

However, this advice doesn't include all people with rheumatoid arthritis. If you have extensive damage to your large joints, high-intensity, weight-bearing exercises may accelerate the progression of joint damage. Instead, try a non-weight-bearing form of exercise such as swimming. Research shows that moderate intensity swimming twice a week in a temperate hydrotherapy pool can significantly improve muscle function in both upper and lower extremities.

HOW MUCH EXERCISE?

People with all forms of arthritis should aim to exercise on at least five days a week – and preferably every day if possible. Your aim should be to start slowly, and gradually work up to a total of 40 minutes exercise a day. You can then start increasing the intensity and/or duration of your exercise program.

You don't have to complete your daily exercise quota in a single session. If it makes it easier, do two or three shorter daily sessions of 10 to 20 minutes each.

Try to base your exercise schedule on the following:

- Do range-of-movement exercises every day to maintain and increase flexibility. This involves putting each joint through its full range of movement by bending, stretching and extending it. I include a stretch routine in the gentle program.
- Do muscle-strengthening exercises, using small weights, every other day to give muscles time to recover.
- Do aerobic exercise at least three times a week – every day if you can.

COPING WITH DISCOMFORT

Pace yourself and respect your limitations when you exercise. Adjust your level of activity to your level of discomfort – if a joint becomes red, swollen or painful, ease off. Learn to listen to your body – if you feel worse the day after exercise, you may have done too much or the activity you've chosen may not be suitable for you. Find ways to minimize pain. Research suggests that some people with arthritis suffer less pain for up to six hours after sex. This may result from increased production of analgesic endorphins in the brain, or from increased secretion of hormones such as testosterone, which have an anti-inflammatory effect. You can also try taking a painkiller before exercise to help relax your muscles and decrease the likelihood of spasm. In addition, you can apply a hot pack to sore joints before exercise – this relieves pain, increases circulation and relaxes muscles. If your joints are painful after exercise, apply an ice pack to them to reduce or prevent swelling and relieve pain.

TYPES OF EXERCISE

Physical activity doesn't need to be vigorous, and it's important to find a type of exercise that you enjoy so that you are motivated to keep it up long term. Even fun activities such as DIY, gardening, dancing and sex count as exercise.

Many people with arthritis are able to enjoy activities that involve weight-bearing such as walking, golf and bowling. You may even be able to do more intensive forms of exercise such as gardening, dancing or jogging. However, if walking is painful, try a less weight-bearing form of exercise such as swimming or cycling (on a recumbent or stationary bike if you prefer). If your arthritis is very advanced, then non-weight-bearing exercise such as cycling or swimming – especially in a hydrotherapy pool (see pages 45–46) – is most appropriate.

WALKING

This is an excellent form of exercise. Suitable for people of all ages and levels of fitness, it is completely free and can easily be incorporated into your daily routine. Get into the habit of leaving the car at home for short, walkable journeys. Invest in a good pair of walking shoes with cushioned soles and some ankle support to protect your feet and lower

EXERCISE AFTER JOINT REPLACEMENT SURGERY

If you've had a hip or knee replacement, your orthopedic surgeon should advise you about which physical activities you can and can't do. When a group of surgeons working for the Mayo Clinic were asked which of several sports they would recommend to their patients following a hip or knee replacement, at least three-quarters agreed that the following activities were ideal: golf, swimming, cycling, sailing, scuba diving and bowling. In addition, they recommended cross-country skiing after a knee replacement. Activities they would not recommend following either a hip or knee replacement included: squash, hockey, handball, baseball/rounders, running, water skiing, karate, basketball, soccer/football and rugby. So, in general, participation in no-impact or low-impact sports is encouraged, but you should avoid participation in high-impact sports.

joints, and consider using a stick (see page 96). When walking, your feet should ideally turn out slightly (15 to 20 degrees) to provide optimum support, and be planted 20 to 25cm (8 to 10in) apart. Keep your knees slightly flexed, and avoid walking on the inner edges of your soles as this makes your ankles rock inward and throws your body out of alignment. Try to keep your head up, your tummy and pelvis tucked in, and your body tilted slightly forward so your weight is on the balls of your feet.

CYCLING

This is a low-impact, non-weight-bearing aerobic activity that, like swimming, doesn't put your muscles, ligaments or joints under excessive strain. You can cycle at home on a stationary bike, in the gym or outdoors. Studies have shown that people who exercise in the fresh air derive greater benefits and get fitter more quickly than those who exercise indoors. Start cycling with a low-gear ratio to keep resistance low. As your stamina increases, introduce more intense bursts of exercise to increase your fitness, if your joints allow. Maintain and oil your bike regularly, and wear a safety helmet made to a recognized standard. Keep to level ground for the first few weeks, then slowly introduce gentle hills, but avoid steep inclines.

SWIMMING

This is a particularly beneficial exercise for arthritis as it involves almost every muscle and joint in your body. The buoyancy of the water supports your weight; and exercising against the resistance of water increases strength, stamina and suppleness. Even just walking through waist-high water is an excellent form of exercise. To get the most benefit from swimming, use a variety of different strokes and swim at least two or three times a week and preferably every day. Consider joining an aqua aerobics class at your local pool. Find out whether there are any hydrotherapy pools in your area – the water is warmer than in standard pools. For safety, never swim alone in case you develop severe pain or spasm while in the water.

GARDENING

This is an excellent form of exercise that can keep you fit and active. If you're already a keen gardener, the following tips will help reduce strain on your joints.

- Don't try to do too much at once – gradually increase the amount of time you spend outdoors.
- Vary your activities – don't spend more than 20 to 30 minutes on each job; plan to do jobs such as digging in stages.
- Use long-handled tools as much as possible to minimize bending or stooping.
- Use a spade and fork that are the right size for you – when buying a tool, go through the motions of planting, raking, digging and so on to make sure the tool fits your build.
- Take only spadefuls of soil that are easy to handle comfortably. By not straining yourself, you will be able to dig for longer.
- Consider installing raised beds and containers so you don't have to stoop so low.
- If you need to be near or on the ground, use a kneeling pad or low stool.
- Don't reach above shoulder level – always use steps.
- Load your wheelbarrow so the weight is mainly over the wheel, and bend your knees, not your back, to lift and lower the barrow.
- When you feel you've had enough or you notice it's starting to get difficult to straighten up, stop.
- Whenever possible, get someone else to do the heavy work for you.

WARMING UP

Whatever form of exercise you do, warming up beforehand is vital to unlock tight muscles and loosen stiff joints. Increasing your body temperature slightly boosts blood-flow to your muscles in preparation for exertion, and reduces the risk of cramp, tearing a muscle or spraining a ligament. Warming up also gets you into the right frame of mind.

Start with several deep breaths, inhaling through your nostrils and exhaling through your mouth. Then spend three to five minutes doing gentle exercises that use the muscles you will need for your exercise. One of the best warming-up exercises is to march on the spot, starting slowly and gradually speeding up. Then start to swing your arms at the same time, at a slow and gentle rate. Now add in some gentle stretches such as a leg stretch (see pages 135–136), hip stretch (see page 134), hamstring stretch (see page 209), shoulder stretch (see page 127) and arm stretch (see pages 123–124).

COOLING DOWN

Cooling down after exercise helps your muscles and joints relax. The cool-down routine is essentially the reverse of your warm-up routine but, as your muscles are still warm and more elastic from your exercise, your muscles gain more benefit from the gentle stretches. Start with the stretches you performed in the warm-up, then finish with light aerobic exercise such as walking, gently marching or jogging on the spot. Cooling down reduces muscle fatigue and soreness, and keeps aches and pains to a minimum later. Both warming up and cooling down enhance flexibility, minimize discomfort, and prevent injury.

MAINTAINING A HEALTHY WEIGHT

Weight loss is one of the most effective ways to reduce pain in your knees and hips, whatever form of arthritis you have. It will also reduce your risk of other health problems such as high blood pressure, raised cholesterol, coronary heart disease, stroke and, possibly, some cancers.

When you walk, the load on your knees increases by four times your body weight. This means that if you are 4.5kg (10lb) overweight, the load on your leg joints is up to 18kg (40lb) more than if you were at a healthy weight. If you are 12.7kg (28lb) overweight, the load on your lower joints is 60kg (112lb) greater than necessary with every step. And that's if you are walking on level ground. When walking downhill, the compressive force on your knees reaches eight times your body weight. This greatly increases the strain on your joints.

But, conversely, if you can lose just 0.45kg (1lb) in weight, there is at least a 1.8kg (4lb) reduction in knee-joint load, which works out at around 2,182kg (4,800lb) per 1.6km (one mile) walked.

The Arthritis Diet and Activity Promotion Trial (ADAPT) confirmed the effectiveness of moderate weight loss achieved through a combination of diet and exercise as a treatment for knee osteoarthritis. Those who combined modest weight loss with moderate exercise enjoyed a 24 percent improvement in their ability to perform daily activities, a reduction in morning stiffness and significant improvements in mobility as well as pain relief. Research shows that weight loss can at least halve the level of pain experienced by people with arthritis affecting their lower limbs – this is a better result than standard drug treatments can achieve.

LOSING WEIGHT

Use the chart on the opposite page to assess whether or not you need to lose any weight. Find your weight in kilograms and draw a line across at that level. Then, find your height in metres and draw a similar line. The point where these two lines meet shows whether you are in the underweight, healthy, overweight, fat or very fat range for your height.

If you're inactive as a result of joint pain, losing weight can be difficult – but not impossible. If you want to lose weight rapidly in the shortest possible time (for the quickest reduction in joint pain), I recommend a very low calorie diet (VLCD) with supervision. This provides less than 800 kilocalories a day. VLCDs typically involve nutritionally complete vitamin- and mineral-enriched drinks and meal replacement products. You can lose an average of 13–23kg (28.6lb–50.6lb) excess weight within a year.

If you don't want to use meal replacement products and you're happy to lose weight over a longer period of time, I recommend a low-glycemic-index diet as your best weight-loss option. This restricts your intake of sugary foods and processed carbohydrates (which cause sharp rises in blood glucose levels, increase insulin secretion and promote fat storage), while still providing the slowly digested complex carbohydrates that are found in many fruits and vegetables. You can lose around 9kg (20lb) after six months on a low glycemic diet. Many GI diet books are available to give guidance about which foods – and how much of them – you can eat.

All of my diet plans in Part Three will also help you to lose some weight – although I haven't designed them as weight-loss programs, the healthy, low-glycemic eating plans should help you to shed weight slowly and naturally. Taking more exercise will also help you lose weight because it increases your metabolic rate and helps you burn more excess fat as a muscle fuel.

YOUR WEIGHT IN KILOS

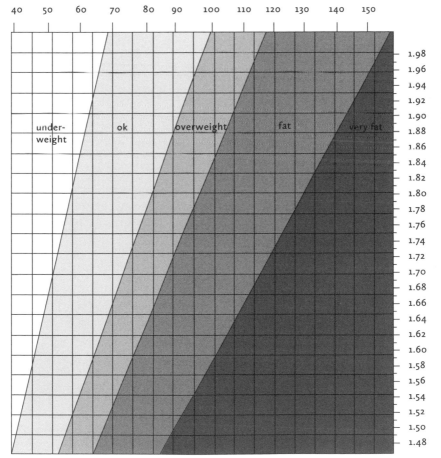

PART THREE

THE NATURAL HEALTH GURU PROGRAMS

Having explained arthritis and the natural approaches to treating it in Parts One and Two, this section of the book provides you with three programs that offer daily practical techniques to overcome arthritis. First, I'd like you to complete a questionnaire that will help to pinpoint the best approach for you: the gentle, moderate or full-strength program. The gentle program is aimed at people with a fair amount of dietary and lifestyle issues to address. It points you in the right direction with a healthy-eating, anti-inflammatory diet that's based around familiar, cosmopolitan dishes. The moderate program is designed for people whose arthritis symptoms are worsened by the chemicals found in foods from the nightshade family of plants (for example, tomatoes, potatoes and bell peppers). Finally, the full-strength program provides an exceptionally high intake of natural antioxidants and anti-inflammatory spices. As well as daily menus, each program provides a nutritional supplement plan, recipes, an exercise routine and complementary therapies to try. Each 14-day program is repeated so the program lasts for 28 days in all. Following one or more of the programs in Part Three should produce significant improvements in your arthritis symptoms.

THE NATURAL HEALTH GURU QUESTIONNAIRE

There are three programs in this section of the book: the gentle, moderate and full-strength programs. There are two ways to approach them: you can do each program sequentially or you can start with the program that seems to best suit your needs.

WORK THROUGH THE PROGRAMS IN SEQUENCE

If you choose to do the programs one by one, the gentle program should be your starting point – this is an antioxidant-rich diet of fruit and vegetables, fish oils, anti-inflammatory spices and other arthritis superfoods. After following the gentle program for a total of one month, you should notice a beneficial effect on your symptoms, in which case it's fine to stay on this program indefinitely. If not, it's possible that your arthritis symptoms are aggravated by the glycoalkaloids present in tomatoes, aubergines, potatoes and chillies (see pages 77–78). I'd therefore like you to move on to the moderate program, which is designed to eliminate these from your diet. If you *are* sensitive to these natural chemicals, a month of the moderate program should produce a marked improvement in your symptoms. If it doesn't, you can move on to the full-strength program. This provides an exceptionally high intake of anti-inflammatory antioxidants plus a number of analgesic spices. If, after following the full-strength program for four weeks, your arthritis symptoms are still not significantly improved, then you may have an idiosyncratic intolerance to some other component of your food intake. On page 76, I explain how to exclude the more common culprits from your diet, then re-introduce them one by one to identify any that appear to trigger your symptoms. You may also wish to consult a naturopath or nutritional therapist who specializes in elimination diets to identify the foods to which you are sensitive.

SELECT THE PROGRAM THAT'S BEST FOR YOU

If you already know or suspect that you're sensitive to the glycoalkaloids present in tomatoes, aubergines, potatoes and chillies, it makes sense to

1 Does arthritis run in your family?
- Don't know   A
- No   A/C
- Yes   C

2 Are your arthritis symptoms worse after eating chillies?
- Don't know   A/B
- Yes   B
- No   A/C

3 How many of your joints are affected by arthritis?
- One or two   A
- Three or four   A/C
- Five or more   C

4 Are your arthritis symptoms worse after eating aubergines?
- Don't know   A/B
- Yes   B
- No   A/C

5 How much pain have you had from your arthritis in the past week?
- Mild   A
- Moderate   A/C
- Severe   C

6 Are your joints very swollen?
- No   A
- A little   A/C
- Yes   C

7 Are your joints very inflamed?
- No   A
- A little   A/C
- Yes   C

8 Do you regularly feel lacking in energy or exhausted?
- Yes, most days   A
- Yes, most weeks   A
- No, not at all   C

9 Are your joints very stiff?
- No   A
- A little   A/C
- Yes   C

10 How often do you eat processed or pre-packaged foods?
- Several times a day   A
- Several times a week   A/C
- Hardly ever   C

11 Do you take regular exercise?
- No   A
- Yes, I walk for 10 minutes three or four times a week   A/C
- Yes, for at least 20 minutes most days   C

12 How often do you eat take-aways?
- Most days   A
- Several times a week   A/C
- Hardly ever   C

13 How often do you eat fried foods?
- Most days   A
- Several times a week   A/C
- Hardly ever   C

14 How many servings of fruit do you usually eat a day?
- One or less   A
- Two   A/C
- Three or more   C

15 Are your arthritis symptoms worse after eating tomatoes?
- Don't know   A/B
- Yes   B
- No   A/C

16 How many servings of vegetables or saladstuff do you usually eat a day?
- One or less   A
- Two   A/C
- Three or more   C

17 How often do you eat fish?
- Hardly ever   A
- Once or twice a week   A/C
- Three or more times a week   C

18 Are you willing to significantly change the way you eat?
- I'll start gently and see how I go   A
- Yes, but without going wild   A/B
- Yes, whatever it takes   B/C

19 Are your arthritis symptoms worse after eating bell peppers?
- Don't know   A/B
- Yes   B
- No   A/C

20 Can you pick up something from the floor?
- Don't know   A
- No   A
- Yes   C

21 Are your arthritis symptoms worse after eating potatoes?
- Don't know   A/B
- Yes   B
- No   A/C

22 Are your symptoms worse after exercise?
- Don't know   A
- No   A/C
- Yes   A

23 Can you reach up to get a heavy object?
- Don't know   A
- No   A
- Yes   C

24 Do you enjoy hot, spicy food?
- As long as it's not too hot   A
- No   A/B
- The hotter the better   C

25 Are you an adventurous eater?
- No, not at all   A
- I try to eat one new dish every week   A/C
- Yes, definitely   C

start on the moderate program straight away. Alternatively, if you have severe pain and swelling, you'll need as many antioxidants as possible in your diet and I would advise starting on the full-strength program. I have also devised the questions on the next two pages to guide you toward the program that's best suited to your needs. When you've completed the questionnaire, work out which response you gave most frequently: A, B or C; and, also, how many Bs or Cs you got.

- If you answered mostly As: start with the gentle program – this is a gentle introduction to a therapeutic diet and it also gets you exercising.
- If you got five or more Bs, start on the moderate program. This excludes plants belonging to the nightshade family; some of your answers suggest these may make your arthritis symptoms worse.
- If you got five or more Cs, start on the full-strength program; your answers suggest that you're prepared for or in need of a high antioxidant diet and an advanced routine of physical stretches.

STARTING THE PROGRAMS

Once you've decided which program you're starting on, read through each day and make a list of the foods, supplements, and any other items you need to purchase – for example, magnetic jewelry (see page 134–135) or a crystal (see page 174). Book appointments with the appropriate complementary therapists, too (see days seven and fourteen of each program).

Whichever program you follow, it's important to monitor your progress. This will give you a clear indication of whether your arthritis symptoms are abating. Take a copy of the following chart and fill it in on the first day of a program and then at seven-day intervals. This chart will also be useful for your doctor to look at when reviewing your medication.

To complete the chart you'll need to assess the severity of your arthritis symptoms using a simple 0 to 10 scoring system. A score of 0 means you have no symptoms, 1 signifies very mild symptoms, 5 means moderate and 10 means the most severe symptoms. It's also useful to include the number of painkillers (for example, paracetamol or ibuprofen) you need to take each day, and your weight.

PROGRESS CHART FOR THE GENTLE, MODERATE AND FULL-STRENGTH PROGRAMS

	DAY OF PROGRAM				
	DAY 1	DAY 7	DAY 14	DAY 21	DAY 28
Date:					
Level of joint swelling (0–10):					
Level of joint stiffness (0–10):					
Level of muscle pain (0–10):					
Level of joint pain (0-10):					
Level of disability (0–10):					
Level of fatigue (0–10):					
Number of painkillers you need a day:					
Weight:					

INTRODUCING THE GENTLE PROGRAM

My aim in the gentle program is to ease you into an arthritis-friendly diet and lifestyle that's simple to follow, yet effective at alleviating joint symptoms. It may take a while to settle into the program, but I'd like you to follow it for at least a month to obtain the full benefits. The program provides 14 daily plans that you can repeat so that it lasts for 28 days altogether. Once you get a feel for the diet and lifestyle changes involved, you can select your own changes to suit your personal likes and dislikes.

THE GENTLE PROGRAM DIET

The diet you'll be following is an omega-3-enriched, anti-inflammatory diet that contains more fish, nuts, seeds, fruit, vegetables, salads and wholegrains than you're probably used to. Olive oil and garlic also play a prominent role. This is a Mediterranean-style diet that is beneficial for "oiling" your joints and reducing pain, swelling and stiffness. It's beneficial for people with all types of arthritis, and can produce significant reductions in pain when followed long term. It's even helpful for people with rheumatoid arthritis, as it decreases disease activity and reduces the risk of heart attack and stroke, to which people with rheumatoid arthritis are known to have an increased susceptibility (see page 17). As a bonus, the Mediterranean way to eat is good for both your immune function and mood regulation.

In addition to Mediterranean flavourings such as garlic, I also include "gentle" spices, such as ginger, for their natural analgesic action.

You can read more about the arthritis superfoods I include in the gentle program on pages 82–86. You may be pleased to know that dark chocolate (choose products that contain at least 70 percent cocoa solids) and a couple of glasses of red wine a week are acceptable treats. Avoid these if they upset your arthritis symptoms, though.

FOODS TO AVOID OR EAT LESS OF

I recommend that you restrict your red meat intake to just two or three times a week – instead of meat for dinner I have included vegetarian or

SHOPPING LIST

These are the items that feature in my suggested menu plans for the next 14 days. Where possible, buy produce regularly for optimum freshness.

DRINKS

apple juice (unsweetened), fruit teas, green, black or white teas, ginger wine, herbal teas (ginger and rosehip), mineral water (low sodium), orange juice (freshly squeezed), wine (red and dry white)

DAIRY PRODUCTS

butter (unsalted), cheese (Cheddar, feta, low-fat goat's, Gruyère, mascarpone, mozzarella, Parmesan and pecorino), ice-cream (low-fat) milk (low-fat semi-skimmed or skimmed), yogurt (low-fat bio)

FRUIT

apples (dessert and cooking), apricots (fresh and dried), bananas, blueberries, cranberries, figs, grapefruit (pink; see caution on page 120), grapes (black, red, green), kiwi fruit, lemons, limes, melon, oranges, peaches, pears, pineapple, plums, pomegranate, raspberries, strawberries, tomatoes

VEGETABLES

avocados, aubergines, bean sprouts, beetroot, bell peppers (red and green), broccoli, butternut squash, carrots, Cos lettuce, courgettes, cucumber, mixed salad leaves, mushrooms (chestnut, mixed wild), onions (red and yellow), parsnips, peas, potatoes, rocket, spinach, spring greens, spring onions, swede, sweetcorn, sweet potatoes, watercress

NUTS AND SEEDS

almonds, Brazils, flax seeds (linseeds), macadamias, pecans, pine nuts, poppy seeds, pumpkin seeds, sesame seeds, sunflower seeds, walnuts

HERBS, SPICES, OILS AND VINEGAR

balsamic vinegar, basil, black pepper, bay leaves, chillies (fresh red and green), cinnamon (ground and sticks), coriander leaf and seeds, cumin, garlic, ginger (powder and fresh), lemongrass, mustard seed, mint, nutmeg, olive oil (standard and extra virgin), oregano, parsley, red wine vinegar, rosemary, star anise, thyme, turmeric, vanilla pod, walnut oil

GRAINS

bread (ciabatta, garlic bread, pitta, and wholemeal bread and rolls), breakfast cereals (high-fibre wheatgerm and wholewheat cereals; instant porridge oats), flour (plain and wholewheat), noodles, pasta (for example, fettuccine, spaghetti and tagliatelle), quinoa, rice (brown)

PROTEINS

eggs (omega-3-enriched), fish (cod, halibut, tuna – fresh and tinned in olive oil – king prawns, salmon and sardines), meat (chicken, lamb fillet, lean beef steak, lean smoked bacon)

MISCELLANEOUS

almond nut milk, caster sugar, cocoa powder, coconut cream, curry paste, dark chocolate (at least 70 percent cocoa solids), filo pastry, fish sauce, ginger wine, honey, mayonnaise (low-fat), olive-oil spread, olives, pesto sauce, soy sauce, sugar (dark brown, Demerara and golden caster), tomato purée, vanilla extract, vegetable bouillon or stock fish dishes on the majority of days. I have excluded added salt, convenience meals and pre-packaged snacks from the gentle program. Convenience and pre-packaged foods, such as ready meals, cakes, biscuits, doughnuts and pastries, contain omega-6 vegetable fats that promote inflammation in the body. Avoiding these foods can significantly help arthritis by increasing your antioxidant consumption and reducing the ratio of your intake of omega-6 oils compared with omega-3s.

Everyone with arthritis is different, and you may find that certain foods I have included in the gentle program seem to worsen your symptoms. If you notice a correlation between your symptoms and eating a particular food, make a point of eliminating that food (be aware of the impact of acid-forming foods; see pages 79–81). If you find that foods from the nightshade family upset your arthritis (tomatoes, potatoes, aubergines, peppers and chillies; see pages 77–78), follow the moderate program instead.

DRINKING PLENTY OF FLUID

Please drink plenty of fluids to help hydrate your joints – especially mineral water that contains good amounts of calcium and magnesium. Keep a small bottle of water with you at all times and take sips regularly throughout the day. Remember that by the time you feel thirsty, you are already significantly dehydrated. Herbal teas such as ginger and rosehip are also beneficial, as are antioxidant-rich black, green and white teas.

LOSING WEIGHT

Although I haven't designed the gentle program as a weight-loss diet, you should find you lose any excess weight slowly and naturally. This is because you're likely to be eating fewer refined carbohydrates and saturated fats than you do normally. These contribute to excess fat, which can worsen arthritis in weight-bearing joints (see pages 103–104). If you need to lose weight, you may wish to enhance the process by eating smaller portions than I suggest in the gentle program and by cutting out some of the starchy foods suggested in each daily plan (for example, wholemeal toast and rolls).

GENTLE PROGRAM SUPPLEMENTS

These are the supplements that I feel are important to take on the gentle program. Take the ones in the recommended list and consider taking some or all of those on the optional list for even more benefits – read pages 87–93 to help you decide. Supplements are widely available in pharmacies, supermarkets and healthfood stores.

Recommended daily supplements
- Vitamin C (500mg)
- Glucosamine sulphate (1,500mg)
- Omega-3 fish oils (1g fish oil capsules, supplying 180mg EPA + 120mg DHA)
- Evening primrose oil (500mg)

Optional daily supplements (these provide additional benefits)
- Vitamin-B complex (25mg)
- Vitamin D (5mcg)
- Vitamin E (200iu/134mg)
- Calcium (500mg)
- Selenium (50mcg)
- Green-lipped mussel extracts (200mg)

THE GENTLE PROGRAM EXERCISE ROUTINE

If you haven't exercised much in recent years, it's important to ease your way gradually into a regular exercise program to avoid aches and pains that may otherwise put you off. I'm going to give you a series of stretch exercises to perform, ideally twice a day, morning and evening. In addition, you should aim to do some brisk aerobic exercise for at least 15 minutes per day.

Walking is one of the easiest and cheapest ways to take aerobic exercise and increase your fitness level. You don't need any special skills or equipment and you can start immediately. I suggest that you buy a small pedometer to clip on to your clothes – this measures the number of steps you take in a day. The optimal number of paces per day for health is 10,000, but this can present a significant challenge when your joints are stiff and painful. I suggest you build up slowly. Start by wearing a pedometer for a few days and simply record the number of steps you take in a day. Don't exert yourself or attempt to increase your level of activity dramatically. Round up the average number of steps you take to the nearest 1,000, then gradually try to increase this by 10 percent. So, for example, if you take 1,000 steps a day, aim to take 1,100 a day over the following week.

Once you are comfortable with a 10 percent increase, make a further 10 percent increase. Keep building up your activity in these gradual stages over the course of your month on the gentle program. As well as increasing the number of steps you take, you can increase the speed at which you walk. However, stop or slow down if you feel you have reached your limit. Here is my suggested walking plan for the gentle program. This will provide a framework within which you can build up your number of daily steps.

- Weeks one and two: walk for 10 minutes a day on Tuesday, Thursday and Saturday.
- Week three: walk for 10 minutes a day on Tuesday and Saturday; and for 15 minutes a day on Thursday and Sunday.
- Weeks four and onward: walk for 15 minutes a day on Tuesday, Thursday, Saturday and Sunday.

THE GENTLE PROGRAM THERAPIES

My aim is to introduce you to some easy-to-follow techniques from some of the less invasive holistic approaches. A number of complementary therapies can help to reduce the pain, swelling and stiffness of arthritis. You can practise some, such as aromatherapy, acupressure, magnetic therapy and meditation, as self-help techniques at home while others are practitioner-led, at least initially. Before you begin the program I suggest that you book an appointment for an aromatherapy massage on day seven of the program, and with a homeopath on day fourteen.

THE GENTLE PROGRAM
DAY ONE

DAILY MENU

Breakfast: Almond Porridge with Fresh Berries (see page 140) **Morning snack:** an apple **Lunch:** bowl of mixed salad leaves with Lemon and Olive Oil Dressing (see the box on page 134) sprinkled with feta cheese, olives, chopped tomatoes, red onions and cucumber. Wholemeal pitta bread. Low-fat bio yogurt with fresh fruit **Afternoon snack:** a handful of walnuts **Dinner:** Cod in Soy Sauce (see page 147). Spinach. Mashed sweet potato. Sweetcorn. Figs in red wine (see page 149) **Drinks:** 570ml/20fl oz/ scant 2⅓ cups semi-skimmed or skimmed milk. Unlimited tea (including herbal or fruit tea) and mineral water **Supplements:** see page 116

I have included apple in every eating plan of the gentle program – either as a mid-morning snack, or as part of your breakfast or dessert menus. Apples are a rich dietary source of anti-inflammatory antioxidants and, as I described on page 82, a fantastic superfood for arthritis.

DAILY EXERCISE ROUTINE

The stretch exercises I show you over the following two weeks will help improve your joint mobility, and strengthen your muscles and bones. Repeat them once or twice a day, adding each day's exercise onto the previous one so you build up a gentle stretch sequence. Start today with a neck stretch.

You may also like to start your walking routine, as outlined on pages 116–117. Walk for at least 10 minutes, three times a week during the first two weeks of the program. If you are already accustomed to walking regularly, then walk for 30 minutes, at least three times per week – and ideally every day. Remember to warm up and cool down (see page 125).

NECK STRETCH

1 Stand comfortably with your feet a little way apart and your shoulders relaxed.

2 Slowly drop your head so your left ear moves toward your left shoulder. Hold the stretch for a count of five. Now repeat on the right-hand side.

AROMATHERAPY

Tonight, I'd like you to place a few drops of lavender essential oil on a tissue or handkerchief and tuck it under your pillow when you go to bed to help you sleep.

DAY TWO

DAILY MENU

Breakfast: bowl of high-fibre cereal. Pink grapefruit (see caution box on page 120) sprinkled with ginger powder **Morning snack:** an apple **Lunch:** Avocado, Mozzarella and Pepper Salad (see page 143). Wholegrain roll. Low-fat bio yogurt with fresh fruit **Afternoon snack:** a handful of macadamia nuts **Dinner:** Mildly Spiced Grilled Chicken (see page 146). Broccoli. Carrots. Brown rice (cook extra for tomorrow's lunch). Strawberries in Balsamic Vinegar with Vanilla Mascarpone (see page 151) **Drinks:** 570ml/20fl oz/ scant 2⅓ cups semi-skimmed or skimmed milk. Unlimited tea (including herbal or fruit tea) and mineral water **Supplements:** see page 116

DAILY EXERCISE ROUTINE

Continue your walking routine, as outlined on pages 116–117. Remember to warm up and cool down. Do yesterday's neck stretch, then add the following shoulder stretch.

SHOULDER STRETCH 1

1 Close your eyes and visualize yourself carrying a heavy briefcase in each hand – let your shoulders be pulled toward the floor.
2 Now imagine dropping the briefcases suddenly. Feel the weight and tension disappear and your shoulders and neck relaxing – your shoulders should move up a little as you do this. Repeat this five times.

AROMATHERAPY

Today, I'd like you to select a single essential oil from those suggested on page 39 (or you can continue to use lavender, or buy a massage oil or lotion from a shop). Add two drops of your chosen oil to 5ml carrier oil and massage into your hands. Rub vigorously to get your hand joints moving.

GRAPEFRUIT – CHECK FOR INTERACTIONS

Today's menu includes grapefruit. If you're taking any medications, check the information leaflet(s) for potential interactions with grapefruit. The bioflavonoids present in grapefruit are beneficial for arthritis, but they can also increase absorption of some drugs. If your drug-insert sheet(s) says you should avoid grapefruit, replace the fruit with an orange – particularly a ruby or blood orange.

DAY THREE

DAILY MENU

Breakfast: Apple, Pineapple and Blueberry Smoothie (see page 140). Wholegrain toast with a scraping of olive-oil spread and honey
Morning snack: a banana
Lunch: Coronation Chicken (see instructions, below). Bowl of brown rice mixed with chopped red pepper and parsley, and drizzled with Lemon and Olive Oil Dressing (see page 134). Low-fat bio yogurt with fresh fruit
Afternoon snack: a handful of walnuts
Dinner: Vegetable Gratinée with Basil and Walnuts (see page 148). Bowl of mixed salad leaves drizzled with olive oil. Crusty garlic bread. A handful of red grapes
Drinks: 570ml/20fl oz/ scant 2⅓ cups semi-skimmed or skimmed milk. Unlimited tea (including herbal or fruit tea) and mineral water
Supplements: see page 116

Today's lunch is coronation chicken. To make it, mix together a handful of chopped fresh apricots with some cooked, shredded chicken breast, a dollop of low-fat mayonnaise and two to three teaspoons of curry paste, (or more or less, if you prefer). Serve the chicken on a bed of lettuce.

DAILY EXERCISE ROUTINE

Continue your walking routine, as outlined on pages 116–117. Remember to warm up and cool down. Do the neck and shoulder exercises from the previous two days of the program, then add the following shoulder stretch to the sequence.

SHOULDER STRETCH 2

1 Move your hands behind your back as if you're going to put them in the back pockets of your trousers – your aim is to move your shoulder blades together and bring your elbows as close together behind your back as you can manage.
2 Relax then repeat five times.

AROMATHERAPY

After massaging your hands as you did yesterday, use your essential oil blend (or a shop-bought massage lotion) to massage any painful joints in your feet as vigorously as you comfortably can. This will warm the joints and stimulate circulation. Now gently move your toes and ankles through their normal range of motion.

DAY FOUR

DAILY MENU

Breakfast: pink grapefruit (see the caution box opposite) sprinkled with ginger powder. Low-fat goat's cheese on a slice of wholegrain bread, drizzled with walnut oil
Morning snack: a pear
Lunch: Chicken, Lime and Grape Salad (see page 143). Wholegrain roll.

Low-fat bio yogurt with fresh fruit
Afternoon snack: a handful of macadamia nuts
Dinner: Thai Salmon Filo Parcels (see page 144). Sweet Chilli Jelly (see page 145). Stir-fried bean sprouts and red peppers. Noodles. Plum, Apple and

Almond Crumble (see page 150)
Drinks: 570ml/20fl oz/ scant 2⅓ cups semi-skimmed or skimmed milk. Unlimited tea (including herbal or fruit tea) and mineral water
Supplements: see page 116

DAILY EXERCISE ROUTINE

Continue your walking routine, as outlined on pages 116–117. Remember to warm up and cool down. Do the stretch exercises from days one to three, then add the following arm stretch.

ARM STRETCH 1

1 Raise your arms above your head. Keep them straight and stretch as high as you can.
2 Lower your arms and let go of tension in your neck, shoulders and arms. Repeat five times.

AROMATHERAPY

Massage your joints with an essential-oil blend or shop-bought massage lotion as on previous days of the program. Then soak your feet in the following essential-oil footbath. If you like, you can substitute your own favourite essential oils for the ones I suggest. If you find the footbath eases pain in your feet, or relaxes you generally, consider investing in a home-spa footbath.

AROMATHERAPY FOOTBATH

1 Add the following essential oils to a bowl of warm water: five drops of lavender, two drops of peppermint and two drops of rosemary.
2 Sit in a comfortable chair with your feet resting in the water. Relax for 15 minutes by reading a book or by closing your eyes and listening to your favourite piece of music.

DON'T OVER-EXERT YOURSELF
Perform your stretch exercises only if you can do so comfortably. If a stretch causes you discomfort, stop.

DAY FIVE

DAILY MENU

Breakfast: Omega-3 Omelette with Tuna and Gruyère (see page 140). Slice of brown bread with a scraping of olive-oil spread
Morning snack: an apple
Lunch: bowl of vegetable soup, for example, carrot and orange (see page 130).

Wholegrain roll. Low-fat bio yogurt with fresh fruit
Afternoon snack: a handful of walnuts
Dinner: Spaghetti Bolognese (use shop-bought sauce or follow your own recipe). Mixed salad. Chocolate Cinnamon Pecan

Brownies (see page 150)
Drinks: 570ml/20fl oz/ scant 2⅓ cups semi-skimmed or skimmed milk. Unlimited tea (including herbal or fruit tea) and mineral water. Glass of red wine (optional)
Supplements: see page 116

Cutting back on the amount of red meat you eat can relieve arthritis symptoms in some people (see page 79). Today, I've included Spaghetti Bolognese for dinner (this will be your first exposure to red meat on the gentle program). Please monitor your joint symptoms carefully over the next one to three days – if you notice that they flare up, this may be a reaction to eating the red meat in the Bolognese. If this is the case for you, I recommend that you avoid meat for the next two weeks. You will need to select a vegetarian meal option in place of the red meat on days eight, nine and fourteen. After two weeks, try reintroducing meat to see if your arthritis flares up again. This elimination and challenge approach is an established way to identify the foods to which you may be intolerant (see page 76).

DAILY EXERCISE ROUTINE

Continue your walking routine (see pages 116–117). Remember to warm up and cool down. Do the stretch exercises from days one to four, then add in the following arm stretch.

ARM STRETCH 2

1 Interlink your fingers and turn your palms outward.

2 Extend your arms in front of you at shoulder height. Hold for 10–20 seconds. Relax, then repeat five times.

HEAT TREATMENT

Prepare some hot compresses as described on page 41. Place hot, wet cloths over your most painful joints. Let the compresses cool to body temperature, then remove. Repeat two or three times. Then, gently move and stretch your joints to help improve their mobility.

DAY SIX

DAILY MENU

Breakfast: Herbed Sardines on Toast (see page 141)
Morning snack: an apple
Lunch: bowl of chopped fresh pineapple, Brazil nuts, grated cheese and mixed salad leaves, drizzled with Lemon and Olive Oil Dressing (see the box on page 134). Wholegrain roll. Low-fat bio yogurt with fresh fruit
Afternoon snack: a handful of macadamia nuts
Dinner: Mushroom and Walnut Roast (see page 149). Spring greens. Chunks of roasted butternut squash or sweet potato. Roast tomatoes. A handful of red grapes
Drinks: 570ml/20fl oz/ scant 2⅓ cups semi-skimmed or skimmed milk. Unlimited tea (including herbal or fruit tea) and mineral water
Supplements: see page 116

Sardines are an excellent source of omega-3 fatty acids. If you don't have time to make the herbed sardines on toast for today's breakfast, then open a tin of sardines or pilchards instead. Those canned in tomato sauce provide additional antioxidants in the form of lycopene – the red tomato carotenoid.

DAILY EXERCISE ROUTINE

Continue your walking routine, as described on pages 116–117. Make sure you warm up and cool down. Do the stretch exercises from days one to five, then add the following finger stretch.

FINGER STRETCH

1 Sit down at a table and rest your hands on the tabletop with your palms facing down. Spread your fingers as wide as you can, and hold the stretch for a count of five.
2 Bring your fingers back together again, while keeping your palms flat on the table. Repeat both steps five times.

AROMATHERAPY

Today's therapeutic treatment is an analgesic aromatherapy bath.

1 Add three drops of lavender and two drops of rosemary essential oils to 15ml carrier oil.
2 Draw your bath so that it is comfortably hot, then add the oils after the taps are turned off. Soak for 15 minutes, ideally in candlelight.

DAY SEVEN

DAILY MENU

Breakfast: a punnet of wild mushrooms sautéed with garlic in a little olive oil. Wholegrain toast
Morning snack: a banana
Lunch: Quinoa, Apricot, Mozzarella and Pomegranate Salad (see page 142). Low-fat bio

yogurt with fresh fruit
Afternoon snack: a handful of walnuts
Dinner: Braised Halibut with Sweet Peppers (see page 148). Broccoli. Sweetcorn. Baked potato. Mulled Cranberry Apples (see page 151)

Drinks: 570ml/20fl oz/ scant 2⅓ cups semi-skimmed or skimmed milk. Unlimited tea (including herbal or fruit tea) and mineral water
Supplements: see page 116

Warming up before aerobic exercise and cooling down afterward is important to maximize joint flexibility and to prevent injury and discomfort. When you go walking, start at a slow speed; then when your joints and muscles have warmed up, you can pick up your pace. You can also use the stretching exercises in this program as warm–ups.

DAILY EXERCISE ROUTINE

Keep up the walking routine outlined on pages 116–117. Remember to warm up and cool down (see page 125). Do the stretch exercises from days one to six, then add this wrist stretch.

WRIST STRETCH

1 Rest your wrists and hands, palms facing down, on a table in front of you. Bend both hands up toward you so you can feel a strong stretch in your wrists. Hold the stretch for a count of five.
2 Turn your hands over so they are resting palms upward. Now bend both hands up toward you again. Hold the stretch for a count of five before relaxing. Repeat each movement five times.

CONSULTING A THERAPIST

Congratulations, you have now been following the gentle program, for one week! By this stage you should have noticed an improvement in your joint symptoms. I now suggest you consolidate these gains by visiting an aromatherapist for a relaxing yet therapeutic aromatherapy massage. An aromatherapist will select essential oils that will help ease painful, stiff joints. A full-body massage lasts around 60 minutes and you will usually feel relaxed afterward. If you enjoy the massage and find that it helps relieve pain and stiffness, book yourself in for a session over each of the next four weeks. To find an aromatherapist, check the resources at the end of this book (see page 234).

DAY EIGHT

Over the next few days I will be introducing you to several different complementary therapies that are beneficial for arthritis. Everyone is different, with different likes and dislikes – once you've found a therapy that suits you, find other ways to incorporate it into your treatment routine. The first complementary technique I'd like you to try is hand reflexology.

DAILY MENU

Breakfast: Almond Porridge with Fresh Berries (see page 140) **Morning snack:** an apple **Lunch:** tuna and sweetcorn salad or sandwich. Bowl of Mixed lettuce leaves drizzled with Lemon and Olive Oil Dressing (see the box on page 134). Low-fat bio yogurt with fresh fruit **Afternoon snack:** a handful of macadamia nuts **Dinner:** Herby Lamb and Aubergine Kebabs (see page 147). Brown rice. Bowl of mixed salad leaves drizzled with Lemon and Olive Oil Dressing (see the box on page 134). Figs in Red Wine (see page 149) **Drinks:** 570ml/20fl oz/ scant 2⅓ cups semi-skimmed or skimmed milk. Unlimited tea (including herbal or fruit tea) and mineral water **Supplements:** see page 116

DAILY EXERCISE ROUTINE

Continue to walk three times a week (or more often if you feel able to), making sure that you warm up and cool down. Perform your routine stretch exercises from days one to seven, then introduce the following shoulder stretch.

SHOULDER STRETCH

1 Stand comfortably with your feet apart. Raise your arms and clasp your hands behind your head. Pull your elbows forward so they are as close together as possible in front of your face. Hold the stretch for a count of five.

2 Now gently swing your elbows out so they are as wide apart as possible. Hold the stretch for a count of five.

HAND REFLEXOLOGY

The underlying principle of reflexology is that parts of your body are represented by "reflexes" on your hands and feet. So massaging the appropriate reflex on your hands or feet can heal the associated body part. Look at the illustrations on page 59 and identify the reflex on your hand that relates to your painful joint or joints. Gently massage the relevant areas on each hand for two minutes. Do this whenever your joints ache.

HUGGING THERAPY
Next time your joint pains start to get you down, indulge in some hugging therapy. Hugging or cuddling someone helps to decrease your perception of pain. This is because hugging triggers the release of oxytocin, a hormone involved in bonding that increases your pain threshold. Hugging a pet works just as well as hugging a human.

DAY NINE

DAILY MENU

Breakfast: plate of fresh fruit: for example, orange, kiwi fruit and grapes. Bowl of high-fibre cereal **Morning snack:** an apple **Lunch:** Avocado and Bacon Salad with Beetroot Mayonnaise (see page 142). Wholegrain roll. Low-fat bio yogurt

with fresh fruit **Afternoon snack:** a handful of walnuts **Dinner:** pasta in pesto sauce. Bowl of mixed salad leaves drizzled with Lemon and Olive Oil Dressing (see the box on page 134). Strawberries in Balsamic Vinegar with

Vanilla Mascarpone (see page 151) **Drinks:** 570ml/20fl oz/ scant 2⅓ cups semi-skimmed or skimmed milk. Unlimited tea (including herbal or fruit tea) and mineral water **Supplements:** see page 116

A high intake of fruit is important when you have arthritis. The antioxidants present in fruit help to reduce inflammation and slow the rate of cartilage breakdown in joints. Today's breakfast gives you a head start.

DAILY EXERCISE ROUTINE
Continue to walk at least three times a week (see pages 116–117). Remember to warm up and cool down. Do the stretch exercises from days one to eight, then add in the following torso stretch.

TORSO STRETCH
1 Stand comfortably with your feet apart and your hands on your hips.

Without moving your lower body, rotate your upper body and hips to the right as far as you can. Hold the stretch for a count of five.

2 Rotate back to the front and repeat toward the left. Repeat five times in each direction.

ACUPRESSURE

Today I recommend you try acupressure to help with your arthritis symptoms. Acupoints around a tender joint often become very sensitive. Press gently around a joint to find the most tender spot and press on it for 10 seconds. Relax and repeat. Do the same on the other side. See the box on page 66 for more on acupressure.

DAY TEN

DAILY MENU

Breakfast: slice of melon. Hard-boiled omega-3-enriched egg. Wholegrain toast with a scraping of olive-oil spread
Morning snack: an apple
Lunch: bowl of vegetable soup such as tomato and basil (see page 130).

Wholegrain roll. Low-fat bio yogurt with fresh fruit
Afternoon snack: a handful of macadamia nuts
Dinner: Mild Prawn and Coconut Curry (see page 145). Brown or red rice. 40–50g (approx 1½oz) bar

dark chocolate (at least 70 percent cocoa solids)
Drinks: 570ml/20fl oz/ scant 2⅓ cups semi-skimmed or skimmed milk. Unlimited tea (including herbal or fruit tea) and mineral water
Supplements: see page 116

The arnica gel you are using today (see page 130) is prepared using the principles of homeopathy and, after immense dilution, contains no measurable amount of arnica. This is different from herbal arnica gel, which contains measurable amounts of the herb (typically from one to 25 percent of *Arnica montana* extract). Make sure you buy a homeopathic version of the gel for the gentle program.

A study involving 172 people with osteoarthritis of the knee compared the use of a homeopathic arnica gel with an NSAID (piroxicam) gel.

Results showed that the homeopathic gel was at least as effective and as well tolerated as the NSAID gel.

DAILY EXERCISE ROUTINE

Continue your walking routine as described on pages 116–117. Remember to warm up and cool down. Do the stretch exercises from days one to nine, then add the following ankle stretch.

ANKLE STRETCH

1 Stand comfortably with your feet slightly apart and one hand resting on the back of a nearby chair or a table for support. Lift both heels up so you are standing on the balls of your feet.
2 Lower your heels down to the floor and relax. Do 10 to 15 complete movements.

HOMEOPATHY

I'd like you to buy a homeopathic preparation of arnica gel to rub into your affected joints. Apply the gel two or three times a day for at least the next five days.

HOME-MADE SOUP

You can easily make a bowl of healthy vegetable soup by gently simmering together any chopped mixed vegetables, tomatoes and herbs in some water or stock. When cooked, purée them in a blender to form a thick, smooth soup – or leave them in chunks if you prefer. Good combinations for soup are tomato and basil, as in today's lunch; carrot and orange; carrot and coriander; leek and potato; and parsnip and apple.

DAY ELEVEN

DAILY MENU

Breakfast: Mediterranean Sauté (see page 141)
Morning snack: a pear
Lunch: chicken salad or sandwich. Low-fat bio yogurt with fresh fruit
Afternoon snack: a

handful of macadamia nuts
Dinner: roast chicken. Roast sweet potato. Spinach. Carrots. Peas. Plum, Apple and Almond Crumble (see page 150)

Drinks: 570ml/20fl oz/ scant 2⅓ cups semi-skimmed or skimmed milk. Unlimited tea (including herbal or fruit tea) and mineral water
Supplements: see page 116

DAILY EXERCISE ROUTINE

Keep up your three-times-a-week walking routine (see pages 116–117), walking further or more frequently as soon as you feel able to. Remember to warm up and cool down. Do the stretch exercises from days one to ten, then do the following hip stretch.

HIP STRETCH 1

1 Stand comfortably with your feet slightly apart and one hand resting on a table for support. Raise your left knee with your leg bent. Bring it up as high in front of you as is comfortable. Feel the stretch in your left hip. Hold for a count of five.

2 Now do the same with the right knee. Repeat the stretch on both sides five times.

HERBALISM

Today, I'd like you to start using a herbal medicine to help your arthritis symptoms. The one I've selected as most appropriate for the gentle program is bromelain, an anti-inflammatory extract from the stems of the pineapple plant (*Ananas comosus*). It can significantly reduce acute knee pain, and stiffness and swelling associated with osteoarthritis and rheumatoid arthritis. It can also reduce pain and bruising after surgery. However, it's not suitable for everyone – you shouldn't take it if you're taking blood-thinning medication, such as aspirin or warfarin, because bromelain also thins the blood. If you want to take it to minimize post-surgical pain and bruising, please check with your surgeon before doing so.

If there is no reason not to take bromelain, start on a 300mg supplement once or twice a day depending on the severity of your symptoms. If you can't take bromelain, consider taking another herb that will help your arthritis – see pages 41–43 for suggestions.

DAY TWELVE

DAILY MENU

Breakfast: porridge swirled with apple purée
Morning snack: a large apple
Lunch: Chicken, Lime and Grape Salad (see page 143). Wholegrain roll. Low-fat bio yogurt with fresh fruit
Afternoon snack: a handful of macadamia nuts

Dinner: vegetarian stew, for example, carrots, tomatoes, squash, swede, courgettes and sweetcorn simmered in vegetable stock with a handful of chopped fresh herbs. Crusty garlic bread. Chocolate Cinnamon Pecan Brownies (see page 150)

Drinks: 570ml/20fl oz/ scant 2⅓ cups semi-skimmed or skimmed milk. Unlimited tea (including herbal or fruit tea) and mineral water. Glass of red wine (optional)
Supplements: see page 116

I have included an optional glass of red wine on days five and twelve of the gentle program. Red wine is a rich source of anti-inflammatory antioxidants, but it doesn't suit everyone. Some people with arthritis find that it can trigger a flare-up of joint pain. If you notice that your arthritis symptoms worsen over the next day or two, and the same thing happened after drinking red wine last week, it's advisable to abstain.

DAILY EXERCISE ROUTINE

Continue your walking routine, as outlined on pages 116–117. Remember to warm up and cool down. Do the stretch exercises from days one to eleven, then do the following hip stretch.

HIP STRETCH 2

1 Stand comfortably with your feet slightly apart and one hand on a table for support. Keep your left leg straight and move it out to the side of your body as far as feels comfortable. Hold for a count of five.
2 Now do the same with the right leg. Repeat on both sides five times.

MEDITATION

This is a simple meditation technique to help reduce joint pain.

COLOUR MEDITATION

1 Sit comfortably in a chair with your eyes shut. Picture a purple colour (purple is healing). Allow it to swirl behind your eyelids. The more colour you can visualize, the stronger the healing effect. If your mind wanders, keep returning to focus on the colour purple.
2 When you feel ready, bring your mind slowly back, open your eyes and enjoy the sense of calm that flows through you. Try to meditate for at least five minutes a day from now on, building up to 15 or more minutes over time.

DAY THIRTEEN

DAILY MENU

Breakfast: Herbed Sardines on Toast (see page 141)
Morning snack: an apple
Lunch: Butternut Squash and Rosemary Pasta (see page 144). Low-fat bio yogurt with fresh fruit

Afternoon snack: a handful of walnuts
Dinner: Mildly Tikka Fish (see page 146). Brown rice. Bowl of mixed salad leaves drizzled with Lemon and Olive Oil Dressing (see page 134). A handful of red grapes

Drinks: 570ml/20fl oz/ scant 2⅓ cups semi-skimmed or skimmed milk. Unlimited tea (including herbal or fruit tea) and mineral water
Supplements: see page 116

Today, I've suggested a cooked lunch of pasta with butternut squash and rosemary. It's quick and easy to make, but if you're short of time, cook fresh pasta in boiling water for three minutes (or follow packet instructions) and stir through some pesto sauce from a jar instead.

DAILY EXERCISE ROUTINE

Continue your walking routine (see pages 116–117). Remember to warm up and cool down. Do the stretch exercises from days one to twelve, then add the following hip stretch.

HIP STRETCH 3

1 Stand comfortably with your feet slightly apart. Put one hand on a table for support.
2 Bend your right knee and lift your right foot up behind you as far as feels comfortable – try to grasp your ankle with your right hand. Your knees should face forward – don't twist them.
3 If you've grasped your ankle, gently ease your foot in toward your right buttock until you feel a mild stretch. Hold for a count of five. Repeat the stretch on your left leg.

MAGNETIC JEWELRY

I'd like you to invest in a piece of magnetic jewelry or an accessory, such as a bracelet, belt, ring, watch or necklace, that you can wear all the time from now on. Magnetic therapy improves circulation and promotes healing in the area where it's worn. In one study of the effects of magnets,

LEMON AND OLIVE OIL DRESSING

Throughout the gentle program I've suggested a simple lemon juice and olive oil dressing to drizzle over your salad. Lemons are rich in vitamin C, and olive oil is an arthritis superfood (see page 85). To make the dressing simply shake 4 tbsp of extra virgin olive oil together with the zest and juice of one large unwaxed lemon. Season with plenty of black pepper.

magnetic patches were found to be 80-percent effective in relieving painful, stiff shoulders, whereas non-magnetized placebos were only six-percent effective.

DAY FOURTEEN

DAILY MENU

Breakfast: pink grapefruit sprinkled with ginger powder (see the caution on page 120). Bowl of high-fibre cereal **Morning snack:** a pear **Lunch:** French Onion Soup (sauté some onions in a little olive oil until caramelized, then add some vegetable or meat stock, heat through and season). Wholegrain roll.

Low-fat bio yogurt with fresh fruit **Afternoon snack:** a handful of macadamia nuts **Dinner:** small steak or chop, marinated in olive oil, garlic and herbs, seasoned with black pepper and grilled. Bowl of mixed salad leaves drizzled with Lemon and Olive Oil Dressing (see

box opposite). Crusty garlic bread. Mulled Cranberry Apples (see page 151) **Drinks:** 570ml/20fl oz/ scant 2⅓ cups semi-skimmed or skimmed milk. Unlimited tea (including herbal or fruit tea) and mineral water **Supplements:** see page 116

DAILY EXERCISE ROUTINE

Continue the walking routine that I described on pages 116–117. From tomorrow start walking on four days a week instead of three (and increase the amount of time you walk by five minutes or more on two of the days). Always warm up before and cool down after your daily walk (or any other form of aerobic exercise). Do the stretch exercises from days one to thirteen, then add the following leg stretch.

LEG STRETCH

1 Lie on a comfortable surface, such as an exercise mat. Bend both knees so your feet are flat on the floor.
2 Lift one leg up in the air and straighten it. Hold for a count of five. Repeat with the other leg. When straightening one leg, always keep the

other knee bent to protect your back. Don't try to lift both legs in the air at the same time.

CONSULTING A HOMEOPATH

Having followed the gentle program for two weeks, you should be experiencing less joint pain and stiffness, and greater mobility. I'd now like you to visit a homeopath. Among 23 people with rheumatoid arthritis, homeopathy significantly improved subjective pain, stiffness and grip strength, while 23 similar people using a placebo showed no significant benefit. A homeopath will choose a remedy specifically for you, based on your symptoms and constitutional type. Homeopaths recognize 15 different constitutional types, based on factors such as your build, personality, likes, dislikes and emotions. Prescribing according to constitutional type is important when treating a long-term condition such as arthritis, for which there are many remedies. To find a homeopath, check the resources on page 235.

MIND YOUR BACK!
Don't do today's exercise if it causes discomfort in your back or if you have back problems. Repeat yesterday's hip stretch instead.

CONTINUING THE GENTLE PROGRAM

Now that you have followed the gentle program for two weeks, I suggest that you repeat the program one more time, so it lasts for 28 days. You can vary the foods you eat, and include some new recipes to introduce variety. You will find some recipe suggestions at www.naturalhealthguru.co.uk and can post your own favourites there, too, for other followers of the program to try.

If you found the gentle program effective in relieving your symptoms and improving your general mobility and well-being, I advise you to stay on it long term. The following information helps you map out your future using the gentle program principles.

YOUR LONG-TERM DIET

The menu plans in the gentle program form part of a healthy, anti-inflammatory diet that encourages consumption of wholegrain foods, fruit, vegetables, salads, low-fat dairy products, fish, nuts and anti-inflammatory spices, such as ginger, chilli and turmeric. The diet also cuts back on your intake of red meat, sugar, saturated fats and salt.

Continue to eat at least five (and preferably eight to 10) servings of fruit, vegetables and saladstuff a day, and aim for a wide range of colours on your plate – the colours in fruit and vegetables are a result of the variety of antioxidant pigments they contain. Check the information on pages 82–86 so you know which are the best superfoods to include in your diet when you have arthritis. Eat a handful of nuts per day, and select wholegrain bread, pasta and cereals rather than processed white versions. Aim to eat two to four portions of fish – especially oily fish – a week if you can (see the box on page 138). If you don't like fish, or are unable to eat it, make sure you take omega-3 fish-oil supplements (see page 91), which are very important for joint health.

Eat red meat only occasionally and, then, have a relatively small serving of 85g/3oz lean meat. Select omega-3-enriched hen's eggs wherever possible as, unlike standard hen's eggs, these have beneficial effects on your blood cholesterol levels. Continue to avoid processed, pre-packaged foods, which tend to contain high amounts of the omega-6 essential fatty acids that are converted into inflammatory substances in the body.

LOSING WEIGHT

If you need to lose weight, cut back on the amount of carbohydrate you eat (for example, bread, rice, pasta and couscous). Aim to eat only as much as you need to feel satisfied – don't feel you have to finish every item on your plate. You can always eat a bit more in an hour or two when you feel hungry again. In fact, having several small meals per day is more beneficial for weight loss than eating larger meals three times a day.

AVOIDING TRIGGER FOODS

If you recognize that certain foods trigger a flare-up in your arthritis symptoms, cut them out of your diet, even if they are recognized arthritis superfoods. Everyone is different and your immune system may have developed an oversensitivity to certain foods. Consult a naturopath or a nutritionist with training in the field of food intolerances to help pinpoint which foods you react against. If you notice that foods from the Solanaceae plant family (for example, tomatoes, potatoes, aubergines and chillies) upset your joint symptoms, you may wish to move onto the moderate program, which eliminates these foods.

YOUR LONG-TERM SUPPLEMENT REGIME

Continue taking the recommended supplements for the gentle program (see page 116) long term if they seem to be working for you. Research supports their use at this level for gentle yet significant effects on joint health. If your joint pain is not yet well controlled, and you are not currently taking all the supplements in the recommended list, you may wish to add in those you have left out. Similarly if, up until now, you have been taking only the supplements in the recommended list, you can add

OILY FISH

Oily fish is an important food in the gentle program diet. All of the following are categorized as oily fish: anchovies, bloater, cacha, carp, eel, herring, hilsa, jack fish, katla, kipper, mackerel, orange roughy, pangas, pilchards, salmon, sardines, sprats, swordfish, trout, tuna (fresh, not tinned) and whitebait. Eat oily fish regularly, but note the advice given in some countries, such as the UK: girls and women who may become pregnant at some time should limit their intake to two portions a week. This is because sea pollutants such as mercury may affect the health of future offspring. Everyone else can eat oily fish up to four times a week.

one or more of the supplements in the optional list. Read pages 87–93 to find out more about the supplements in which you are interested.

YOUR EXERCISE ROUTINE

After two weeks of regular joint stretching exercises, you should have started to notice an increase in flexibility. Continue to do these stretch exercises, ideally twice a day. If you feel able to do more, try the stretch exercises in the moderate program.

You should also be sure to maintain your aerobic exercise routine. When you reached the third week of the gentle program you should have started to walk on four days a week instead of three (see pages 116–117). If you're already walking more frequently and for a longer duration than I suggest in the schedule on page 117, that's great – just keep increasing the number of paces you take each day and stop when you feel that you've reached a comfortable limit. If you want a change from walking, try other activities such as cycling, swimming, dancing, gardening, bowling and golf – whatever activities you like doing and which your joints allow you to do.

YOUR THERAPY PROGRAM

The gentle program has shown you how to use aromatherapy and other techniques such as magnetic therapy, homeopathy, herbal medicine and meditation. If you found their treatments useful, continue to consult the natural healthcare professionals – the aromatherapist and homeopath – I suggested you find on days seven and fourteen.

MONITORING YOUR JOINT SYMPTOMS

While continuing on the gentle program I suggest you monitor and score your joint symptoms on a weekly basis. This will enable you to see whether you are continuing to benefit from the program. If your joint scores stop improving, or if they start to worsen again, I suggest you increase the level of supplements you take to that suggested for the moderate program (see page 156). You may also wish to move onto the moderate program.

BREAKFAST RECIPES

ALMOND PORRIDGE WITH FRESH BERRIES

SERVES 4

600ml/21fl oz/scant 2½ cups almond
    nut milk
150g/5½oz/½ cup porridge oats
¼ tsp freshly ground cinnamon
1 handful flaked almonds
1 handful fresh berries

1 Bring the milk just to boiling point
   in a saucepan. Add the porridge oats
   and cinnamon. Simmer gently for
   1 minute (or follow the instructions
   on the packet) while stirring.

2 Remove from the heat, cover and
   stand for at least 5 minutes until all
   the liquid is absorbed. Sprinkle the
   almonds and berries on top and serve.

APPLE, PINEAPPLE AND BLUEBERRY SMOOTHIE

SERVES 4

400g/14oz/heaped 2⅓ cups porridge oats
1 red eating apple, cored
1 pineapple, peeled, cored and cut into
    chunks
1 handful blueberries
100ml/3½fl oz/scant ½ cup unsweetened
    apple juice

1 Put the ingredients in a food
   processor and blend until smooth.
   Add more or less apple juice if you
   prefer a lighter or thicker smoothie.

OMEGA-3 OMELETTE WITH TUNA AND GRUYÈRE

SERVES 4

8 omega-3-enriched eggs
2 tbsp olive oil
1 handful grated Gruyère cheese
185g/6½ oz can flaked tuna in olive oil,
    drained
1 handful chopped parsley
Freshly ground black pepper

1 Beat the eggs lightly and season with
   plenty of black pepper.

2 Heat the olive oil in a large non-stick
   pan over high heat. Tip in the eggs
   and gather the curds into the middle
   as the egg sets.

3 When there is only a little runny egg
   left, remove from the heat. Scatter
   the Gruyère and tuna over one half
   of the omelette. Season with more
   black pepper.

4 Return to the heat and warm through
   for 30 seconds. Flip the uncovered
   side of the omelette over. Slide out
   onto a plate, sprinkle with parsley
   and serve.

HERBED SARDINES ON TOAST

SERVES 4

4 fresh sardines, cleaned
2 tbsp olive oil
1 small red onion, sliced
1 handful chopped herbs, for example,
   oregano, thyme, rosemary, basil
   and parsley
1 garlic clove, crushed
8 cherry tomatoes, halved
Zest and juice of ½ unwaxed lemon
4 slices wholegrain bread, toasted
Freshly ground black pepper

1 Brush the sardines with olive oil and
   sauté them with the onion, herbs and
   garlic until they start to turn golden.

2 Add the tomatoes and lemon zest
   and juice and simmer gently for 5
   minutes or until cooked through.

3 Put the sardine mixture on the slices
   of toast, season well with black
   pepper and serve.

MEDITERRANEAN SAUTÉ

SERVES 4

4 tbsp olive oil
1 red onion, sliced
1 garlic clove, crushed
1 handful chopped herbs, for example,
   oregano, thyme, rosemary, basil and
   parsley
4 mushrooms, chopped
8 cherry tomatoes, halved
2 small courgettes, chopped
1 red pepper, deseeded and cut
   into strips
1 green pepper, deseeded and cut
   into strips
1 baby aubergine, chopped
4 slices wholegrain bread, toasted
Freshly ground black pepper

1 Heat the olive oil in a pan and sauté
   the red onion, garlic and herbs for
   2 minutes. Add the remaining
   vegetables and sauté for a further 5
   minutes or until cooked to your liking.

2 Put the vegetables on the slices of
   toast, season well with black pepper
   and serve.

LUNCH RECIPES

QUINOA, APRICOT, MOZZARELLA AND POMEGRANATE SALAD

SERVES 4

200g/7oz/1 heaped cup quinoa
8 semi-dried apricots, chopped
1 handful mixed seeds, for example,
    pumpkin, sesame, sunflower, poppy,
    flax seeds (linseeds) and pine nuts
1 pomegranate
2 buffalo mozzarella balls, chopped
1 handful chopped coriander leaves
4 handfuls mixed lettuce leaves
Freshly ground black pepper

1 Cook the quinoa according to the packet instructions, then drain and rinse it. Put it in the fridge to chill.

2 Halve the pomegranate and, holding each half over a large bowl, bash the outer skin with a wooden spoon until all the seeds fall out into the bowl. Mix together with the chilled quinoa and all the other remaining ingredients, except the lettuce and pepper. Season well with black pepper, put on top of the lettuce and serve.

AVOCADO AND BACON SALAD WITH BEETROOT MAYONNAISE

SERVES 4

6 slices lean, smoked bacon
2 avocados, peeled, stoned and sliced
Zest and juice of 1 unwaxed lemon
12 cherry tomatoes, halved
4 spring onions, chopped
½ cucumber, chopped
100g/3½oz pecorino cheese,
    sliced thinly
4 handfuls mixed baby salad leaves
Freshly ground black pepper

For the beetroot mayonnaise:
1 small beetroot, unpeeled
100ml/3½fl oz/scant ½ cup low-fat
    mayonnaise
1 tbsp red wine vinegar

1 Grill the bacon until crispy. Leave it to cool, then break it into small pieces.

2 Mix the avocado with the lemon zest and juice. Add the bacon and other salad ingredients and season well.

3 Boil the beetroot in water until cooked. Peel then blend the beetroot with the mayonnaise in a blender. Add the red wine vinegar. Serve the salad with the beetroot mayonnaise.

AVOCADO, MOZZARELLA AND PEPPER SALAD

SERVES 4

2 avocados, peeled, stoned and sliced
Zest and juice of 1 unwaxed lemon
1 red pepper, deseeded and chopped
1 handful torn basil leaves
125g/4½oz mini mozzarella balls
1 handful walnuts, chopped
4 tbsp walnut oil
1 ciabatta, sliced and toasted
Freshly ground black pepper

1 Mix the avocado slices with the lemon zest and juice to prevent discoloration. Add the red pepper, basil, mozzarella, walnuts and walnut oil and leave to infuse for 30 minutes.

2 Put the salad on the ciabatta slices, season with black pepper and serve.

CHICKEN, LIME AND GRAPE SALAD

SERVES 4

4 chicken breasts
2 tbsp olive oil
Zest and juice of 4 unwaxed limes
1 red onion, finely chopped
1 garlic clove, crushed
2 tbsp fish sauce
1 tbsp caster sugar
1 cos lettuce, chopped
175g/6oz red grapes
A few sprigs mint, chopped
Freshly ground black pepper

1 Preheat the oven to 200°C/400°F/ Gas 6. Brush the chicken with some of the olive oil and half the lime juice. Roast for 20 minutes until cooked.

2 Heat the remaining oil in a pan and sauté the onion and garlic until soft. Add the remaining lime juice, and the zest, fish sauce and sugar.

3 Toss the lettuce leaves and grapes in the sauce. Put the chicken on top of the lettuce, pour the sauce over, season with black pepper, sprinkle with the mint and serve.

DINNER RECIPES

BUTTERNUT SQUASH AND ROSEMARY PASTA

SERVES 4

450g/1lb fresh pasta or 350g/12oz
  dried pasta
85g/3oz unsalted butter
2 garlic cloves, crushed
450g/1lb butternut squash, peeled,
  deseeded and cut into bite-sized
  pieces
5 sprigs rosemary, finely chopped
Zest and juice of 1 unwaxed lemon
¼ tsp freshly ground nutmeg
55g/2oz/½ cup fresh Parmesan cheese,
  shaved
Freshly ground black pepper

1 Cook the pasta according to the
  instructions then drain.

2 Melt the butter in a pan and sauté
  the garlic for 30 seconds, before
  adding the butternut squash, the
  chopped leaves of 1 rosemary sprig
  and the lemon zest and juice. Cover
  and sweat over a gentle heat for
  15 minutes, stirring occasionally.

3 Mash half the squash into the butter.
  Season with black pepper and
  nutmeg. Mix with the pasta and
  sprinkle the remaining rosemary
  and the Parmesan on top. Serve.

THAI SALMON FILO PARCELS

SERVES 4

4 salmon fillet steaks
4 sheets ready-rolled filo pastry
4 tbsp Sweet Chilli Jelly (see following
  recipe)
55g/2oz butter, melted

1 Preheat the oven to 200°C/400°F/
  Gas 6. Put a fillet of salmon at the
  end of each piece of filo pastry. Use
  some of the Sweet Chilli Jelly to coat
  the fish.

2 Brush the surrounding filo pastry
  with some of the melted butter and
  wrap up the salmon, folding the sides
  in to make a parcel. Repeat with the
  remaining pieces of salmon.

3 Brush the tops of the parcels
  with melted butter and bake for
  20 minutes. Serve with the remaining
  Sweet Chilli Jelly.

SWEET CHILLI JELLY

MAKES 425G/1LB

3 cooking apples, chopped (include the
   cores, peel and pips)
1 handful fresh or frozen cranberries
2 fresh red chillies, finely chopped
½ red pepper, deseeded and chopped
200ml/7fl oz/⅘ cup red wine vinegar
175g/6oz/scant 1 cup caster sugar

1 Put all the ingredients (except the
   sugar) and 200ml/7fl oz/ scant 1 cup
   water in a pan, bring to the boil and
   simmer gently for 20 minutes, stirring
   occasionally. Allow to cool slightly,
   then mash the apple pieces, adding
   more water if necessary to obtain
   a slightly runny sauce.

2 Sieve the sauce or drain it through a
   muslin cloth suspended over a large
   bowl (this may take several hours).
   Pour more water through the pulp,
   if necessary, so you end up with
   250ml/9fl oz/1 cup of juice.

3 To make the jam, heat the juice with
   the sugar, stirring continuously until
   the sugar dissolves. Bring to the boil
   and simmer gently – skimming off
   any scum – for 10 minutes. Put a
   teaspoon of the jam on a cold plate
   and, when cool, press with a finger:
   if the surface wrinkles, the jelly is set.
   Remove from the heat, skim, allow to
   cool and then pour into a clean, dry
   425g/1lb jar.

MILD PRAWN AND COCONUT CURRY

SERVES 4

2 tbsp olive oil
2 tsp mustard seeds
1 onion, finely chopped
2½cm/1in piece root ginger, peeled
   and finely chopped
2 garlic cloves, crushed
½ tsp turmeric
1 tsp ground coriander
2 bay leaves
1–2 fresh green chillies, finely sliced
   (deseed for gentler heat)
20 raw king prawns, peeled
400ml/14fl oz/1½ cups coconut cream
Zest and juice of 2 unwaxed limes
1 handful chopped coriander

1 Heat the oil in a pan and sauté the
   mustard seeds for 30 seconds. Add
   the onion and cook until soft. Add
   the ginger, garlic, turmeric and
   coriander and stir-fry for 1 minute.

2 Add the bay leaves, chillies and
   300ml/10½fl oz/scant 1¼ cups
   water and bring to the boil. Simmer
   gently for 1 minute before adding
   the prawns. Simmer for a further
   4 minutes until the prawns are
   cooked, then add the coconut cream,
   lime zest and juice and coriander.
   Warm through and serve.

MILDLY TIKKA FISH

SERVES 4

2½cm/1in piece root ginger, peeled and
    finely chopped
4 garlic cloves, crushed
100ml/3½fl oz/scant ½ cup low-fat
    bio yogurt
2 tbsp olive oil
2 tsp turmeric
1 fresh red chilli, deseeded and finely
    chopped
2 tsp cumin seeds
4 fish steaks, for example, tuna

1 Make the tikka mixture by mixing all
    the ingredients except the fish steaks
    together. Coat the fish in the tikka
    mixture and then leave to marinate
    in the fridge for at least 2 hours.

2 Grill or barbecue the fish for
    4 minutes per side or until just
    cooked through.

MILDLY SPICED GRILLED CHICKEN

SERVES 4

4 chicken breasts

For the marinade:
1 fresh red chilli, deseeded and chopped
1 onion, chopped
1 lemongrass stalk, trimmed and
    chopped
4 tbsp olive oil
2 tsp dark brown sugar
Juice and zest of 1 unwaxed lemon
½ tsp turmeric

1 Score the chicken breasts.

2 Put the marinade ingredients in a
    blender and blend to make a paste.
    Coat the chicken with the paste and
    leave to marinate in the fridge for at
    least 2 hours.

3 Barbecue or grill the chicken on
    a high heat until it is cooked.

HERBY LAMB AND AUBERGINE KEBABS

SERVES 4

450g/1lb lean fillet of lamb, cubed
1 aubergine, cut into cubes

For the marinade:
4 tbsp olive oil
Zest and juice of 1 unwaxed lemon
2 garlic cloves, crushed
1 sprig rosemary, chopped
4 sprigs thyme, chopped
Freshly ground black pepper

1 Mix together the marinade
   ingredients, season with black pepper
   and pour over the lamb and aubergine.
   Marinate for at least 1 hour.

2 Thread the lamb and aubergine
   alternately onto 8 skewers, then
   barbecue or grill on a high heat to
   seal the meat. Reduce the heat and
   cook for 10 minutes, basting and
   turning frequently.

COD IN SOY SAUCE

SERVES 4

4 tbsp olive oil
1 red onion, finely chopped
2 garlic cloves, crushed
1 fresh red chilli, deseeded and chopped
   (optional)
2½cm/1in piece root ginger, peeled and
   finely chopped
4 cod fillets
2 tomatoes, skinned and chopped
Zest and juice of 1 small unwaxed lemon
2 tbsp dark soy sauce
1 tbsp dark brown sugar
½ cucumber, thinly sliced
1 handful chopped parsley

1 Heat the olive oil in a pan and sauté
   the onion and garlic until soft. Add
   the chilli and ginger.

2 Add the fish followed by the
   tomatoes, lemon zest and juice, soy
   sauce and sugar. Simmer until the fish
   is cooked.

3 Put the fish on the cucumber, pour
   the sauce over the top and sprinkle
   with parsley.

BRAISED HALIBUT WITH SWEET PEPPERS

SERVES 4

3 red peppers, halved and deseeded
3 yellow peppers, halved and deseeded
6 garlic cloves
3 sprigs thyme
3 sprigs rosemary
1 handful chopped basil leaves
80ml/2½fl oz olive oil
4 halibut fillets
125ml/4fl oz/½ cup vegetable stock
1 handful chopped parsley
Freshly ground black pepper

1 Preheat the oven to 200°C/400°F/Gas 6.

2 Put the pepper halves face down on a baking sheet. Sprinkle the garlic, thyme and rosemary over the top and bake for around 25 minutes, until the pepper skins start to blister.

3 Put the peppers in a bowl (discard the garlic and herbs) and cover with cling-film to make peeling easier. When cool, peel the peppers and cut into strips.

4 Sauté the peppers with the basil and half the oil for 3 minutes. Season well with black pepper and keep warm.

5 Shallow-fry the halibut with the remaining olive oil (skin-side down) for 5 minutes until coloured. Turn over and cover with the stock. Simmer for 5 minutes until cooked through.

6 Put the fish on top of the peppers and season well. Sprinkle the parsley over the top and serve.

VEGETABLE GRATINÉE WITH BASIL AND WALNUTS

SERVES 4

4 tbsp olive oil
2 medium aubergines, cut into slices lengthways
4 courgettes, sliced lengthways
450g/1lb baby spinach leaves, chopped
2 handfuls walnuts, coarsely chopped
115g/4oz mozzarella or Cheddar cheese, grated
30g/1oz/⅓ cup grated Parmesan

For the sauce:
6 tomatoes, chopped
1 red pepper, deseeded and chopped
2 tbsp olive oil
1 onion, chopped
2 garlic cloves, crushed
1 tbsp tomato purée
1 handful chopped basil
100ml/3½fl oz/scant ½ cup dry white wine
Freshly ground black pepper

1 Preheat the oven to 190°C/375°F/Gas 5.

2 Lightly brush a heavy pan with olive oil and fry the aubergine and courgette slices until they start to colour. Drain on absorbent paper.

3 Steam the spinach leaves until just wilted. Drain.

4 To make the sauce, purée the tomatoes and red pepper in a blender. Heat the olive oil in a pan and sauté the onion and garlic. Add the tomatoes, red pepper, tomato purée, basil and white wine. Bring to the boil and simmer, stirring, until

starting to thicken. Season well with black pepper.

5 Place alternating layers of aubergine and courgette slices, sauce and spinach in an ovenproof dish. Top with the walnuts and grated cheese and bake for 30 minutes.

MUSHROOM AND WALNUT ROAST

SERVES 4

2 tbsp olive oil
1 onion, finely chopped
2 garlic cloves, crushed
8 chestnut or brown cap mushrooms, chopped
225g/8oz/2 cups walnuts finely chopped
115g/4oz fresh wholemeal breadcrumbs
1 omega-3-enriched egg, beaten
3 parsnips, peeled, boiled and mashed
4 tbsp low-fat bio yogurt
1 handful chopped mixed herbs, for example, basil, thyme, rosemary and parsley
150ml/5fl oz/scant ⅔ cup vegetable stock
Freshly ground black pepper

1 Heat the oven to 180°C/350°F/Gas 4.
2 Lightly brush a large loaf tin with oil. Put the remaining oil in a pan and sauté the onion, garlic and

mushrooms. Mix together the walnuts, breadcrumbs and egg.

3 Mash the parsnips with the yogurt and herbs. Add the egg, mushroom mix and stock, and season with black pepper.

4 Put in the loaf tin, cover with foil and bake for 50 minutes. Leave to stand for 10 minutes before turning out.

DESSERT RECIPES

FIGS IN RED WINE

SERVES 4

200g/7oz/1 cup plus 1 tbsp golden caster sugar
200ml/7fl oz/scant 1 cup red wine
8 firm but ripe figs, peeled

1 Put the sugar, 400ml/14 fl oz/1½ cups water and the wine in a pan and gently bring to a simmer, stirring until the sugar dissolves. Add the figs, cover and poach gently for 8 minutes.

2 Remove the figs with a slotted spoon and allow to cool. Continue to simmer the syrup for 15 minutes to reduce the volume. Allow to cool slightly, then pour over the figs. Serve warm.

CHOCOLATE CINNAMON PECAN BROWNIES

SERVES 4

100g/3½oz dark chocolate (70 percent
cocoa solids)
125g/4½oz unsalted butter (softened
at room temperature)
275g/9¾oz/1¼ cups caster sugar
1 tsp vanilla extract
2 eggs, beaten
85g/3oz/⅔ cup plain flour
4 tbsp cocoa powder
1 tsp ground cinnamon
100g/3½oz pecan nuts, chopped

1 Preheat the oven to 180°C/350°F/Gas 4.

2 Gently melt the chocolate in a
   heatproof bowl over a pan of
   simmering water.

3 Beat the butter until soft and creamy.
   Add the sugar and vanilla extract and
   beat until fluffy. Gradually beat in the
   eggs, then sift over the plain flour,
   cocoa powder and cinnamon. Add the
   pecan nuts and melted chocolate and
   stir gently until thoroughly mixed.

4 Pour into a non-stick 20cm/8in square
   cake tin. Bake for 30 minutes. Cut into
   squares and serve warm.

PLUM, APPLE AND ALMOND CRUMBLE

SERVES 4

400g/14oz dark red or black plums,
stoned and chopped
2 Red Delicious apples, cored and
chopped
1 tsp ground cinnamon
1 tsp soft brown sugar (optional)

For the crumble topping:
85g/3oz/⅔ cup wholemeal flour
30g/1oz butter
1 tsp ground cinnamon
55g/2oz/¼ cup Demerara sugar
55g/2oz/⅓ cup almonds, chopped

1 Preheat the oven to 200°C/400°F/
   Gas 6.

2 Mix all the filling ingredients together
   and put in an ovenproof dish.

3 Rub the flour and butter together in
   a bowl with your fingers, then stir
   in the cinnamon, sugar and almonds.

4 Sprinkle the crumble topping over
   the fruit and press down firmly.
   Bake for 40 minutes. Allow to rest
   for 15 minutes before serving warm.

STRAWBERRIES IN BALSAMIC VINEGAR WITH VANILLA MASCARPONE

SERVES 4

600g/1lb 5oz strawberries, washed, hulled and halved
150ml/5fl oz/⅔ cup aged balsamic vinegar
5 tbsp dark brown sugar
1 vanilla pod
400g/14oz mascarpone cheese
1 handful chopped mint leaves, chopped

1 Put the strawberries, balsamic vinegar and dark brown sugar in a bowl and mix. Leave the fruit to marinate for 1 hour, stirring regularly.

2 Score the centre of the vanilla pod and scrape out the seeds (tip: put the scraped vanilla pod in a jar and cover with golden caster sugar to make vanilla-flavoured sugar – you can use this to sprinkle over ripe strawberries in the future). Mix the seeds with the mascarpone cheese and leave to infuse.

3 Serve the strawberries and mascarpone with the mint sprinkled on top.

MULLED CRANBERRY APPLES

SERVES 4

250ml/9fl oz/1 cup freshly squeezed orange juice
6 tbsp ginger wine
2½cm/1in piece root ginger, peeled and chopped
1 cinnamon stick
1 star anise
4 red apples, cored and chopped
2 handfuls fresh or frozen cranberries
2 tbsp golden caster sugar
Low-fat ice cream, to serve

1 Put all the ingredients in a pan and bring to the boil, stirring until the sugar dissolves. Simmer gently for 5 minutes, then remove from the heat and allow to cool.

2 Remove the star anise and cinnamon stick and serve with the ice cream.

INTRODUCING THE MODERATE PROGRAM

The moderate program is a more advanced dietary and lifestyle plan for arthritis than the gentle program. It's designed for people whose joint pain, stiffness and swelling remain troublesome, despite eating plenty of oily fish, nuts, fruit and vegetables. One of the key features of the moderate program is that it will help you recognize whether or not your symptoms are worsened by eating foods from the nightshade family of plants (see chart opposite).

THE MODERATE PROGRAM DIET

The diet eliminates the foods from the nightshade family, as well as foods made with these foods, such as tomato ketchup, tomato purée and Tabasco sauce. As described on pages 77–78, these foods contain substances known as glycoalkaloids, which can worsen muscle and joint pain in some people (the reason for this is not fully understood). Some research suggests that eliminating nightshade plants from the diet can improve symptoms in 10 percent of people with arthritis of various types – others suggest it can help as many as 70 percent of people with arthritis.

EAT FRUIT, VEGETABLES, NUTS AND FISH

The moderate program diet contains plenty of non-nightshade fruit and vegetables that are rich in antioxidants, vitamins and minerals. In particular, I encourage you to drink apple juice and to eat fish, apples, Brazil nuts (for their rich selenium content) and macadamia nuts. With a delicious mild, crunchy flavour, macadamias contain as much as 75 percent oil, which has the highest content of monounsaturated fat found anywhere in nature.

DESSERT RECIPES

Some of the dessert recipes are more decadent than usually found in my Natural Health Guru books. For example, cinnamon chocolate nut terrine (see page 190) includes double cream and sugar, and the raspberry and red wine sorbet (see page 190) includes red wine and sugar. This is

MEMBERS OF THE NIGHTSHADE (SOLANACEAE) FAMILY

FOOD	BOTANICAL NAME
Aubergine	*Solanum melongena*
Bell peppers	*Capsicum annuum*
Cape gooseberry (ground cherry)	*Physalis peruviana, P. ixocarpa*
Garden huckleberry	*Solanum melanocerasum*
Habanero peppers	*Capsicum chinense*
Naranjillas	*Solanum quitoense*
Paprika/chilli powder	*Capsicum annuum* (dried)
Pepinos	*Solanum muricatum*
Potato	*Solanum tuberosum*
Tabasco peppers	*Capsicum frutescens*
Tamarillo	*Solanum betaceum*
Tomatillo	*Physalis philadelphica*
Tomato	*Solanum esculentum / Lycopersicon esculentum*
Tobacco	*Nicotiana tabacum* (see page 96 for advice on quitting smoking)

justified during the moderate program in that, nutritionally, the other ingredients are extremely healthy. (Also, red wine and dark chocolate are rich in antioxidants.) My primary aim is simply to test whether or not your problems are linked to the consumption of nightshade glycoalkaloids. If you prefer to omit cream, sugar and alcohol from your diet, replace richer dishes with fruit or eat 40–50g (approximately 1½oz) plain dark chocolate (at least 70 percent cocoa solids) by itself.

DRINKING PLENTY OF FLUIDS

As with all the programs, you need to drink plenty of fluids to hydrate your joints. Keep a small bottle of water or cold herbal tea (for example, ginger tea) with you and sip it regularly throughout the day. Drink more in hot climates or when you are more active than usual (for example, during or after your daily exercise routine). Remember that by the time you feel thirsty, you are already dehydrated.

SHOPPING LIST

This list shows you the non-nightshade foods you can eat on the moderate program.
Base your shopping lists on these items, which feature in the recipes and eating plans.

DRINKS

apple juice (unsweetened), fruit teas, green, black or white teas, herbal teas, mineral water (low sodium), wine (red and dry white)

DAIRY PRODUCTS

butter (unsalted), crème fraîche, double cream, fromage frais (low-fat plain and vanilla), milk (low-fat semi-skimmed or skimmed), yogurt (plain low-fat bio and Greek yogurt); cheeses: Cheddar, cottage cheese (plain, with chives, pineapple), dolcelatte, Gorgonzola, haloumi, mozzarella, Parmesan, pecorino, Roquefort, Stilton (select low-fat versions)

FRUIT

apples (especially Red Delicious and cooking), apricots (fresh and semi-dried), bananas, blackberries, blueberries, dates, figs (fresh and dried), grapefruit (blond, pink, red; see caution on page 120), grapes (green, red, black), guava, kiwi fruit, lemons, mango, oranges, papaya, peaches, pears, pineapple, plums, pomegranate, prunes, raisins, raspberries, strawberries, watermelon

VEGETABLES

avocados, bean sprouts, beetroot, black beans, broccoli, butternut squash, cabbage (red and green), carrots, celery, celeriac, chickpeas, courgettes, cucumber, Florence fennel, green beans, lentils (red, green), mixed salad leaves, mushrooms, onions (baby, white, red), pumpkin, radish, rocket, spinach, spring onions, sprouted beans, sweetcorn, sweet potatoes, watercress

NUTS AND SEEDS

almonds, hazelnuts, macadamias, pecans, pistachios, pumpkin seeds, sesame seeds, walnuts

HERBS, SPICES, OILS AND VINEGAR

basil, bay leaves, black pepper (freshly ground), chives, cinnamon (sticks and ground), cloves (whole and ground), coriander (leaves and seeds), cumin, dill, fennel, garlic, mint, nutmeg, oregano/marjoram, parsley, peppercorns (black, green, red), rosemary, sage, tarragon, thyme, turmeric; extra virgin olive oil (for drizzling and dressings), olive oil (for cooking), macadamia nut oil, walnut oil; red wine vinegar, white wine vinegar

GRAINS

coarse oatmeal, fresh and dried pasta (wholemeal and hemp), muesli (unsweetened), high-fibre breakfast cereals, porridge oats, wholegrain/multigrain bread and rolls, speciality breads (ciabatta and focaccia), rye bread, wholemeal pitta bread, rice (brown, red, risotto and wild), rice noodles, rolled oats, quinoa, wheatflour (plain) or similar, wholemeal bread

PROTEINS

omega-3-enriched eggs; fish: anchovy, bream, haddock (smoked, no colourings), herrings, mackerel, mullet (grey), prawns, salmon (fresh and smoked), red snapper, sea bass, trout (fresh and smoked), tuna (fresh and tinned in olive oil); meat: bacon (lean), chicken, pork chops

MISCELLANEOUS

bouillon cubes (beef, chicken or vegetable), black olives, dark chocolate (70 percent cocoa solids), hummus, mayonnaise, mustard (wholegrain), olive-oil spread, runny honey, sugar (caster and golden caster, and dark and soft brown), vanilla extract

LOSING WEIGHT

Although the moderate program is not designed for weight loss, you should find that you will lose any excess weight slowly and naturally as a result of eating healthily. If you need to lose weight, you can accelerate the process by eating smaller portions, especially of starchy foods, such as pasta, bread and rice. Also, omit the dessert recipes that include sugar and cream.

THE MODERATE PROGRAM EXERCISE ROUTINE

The exercise program provides you with a series of stretches that will improve your joint flexibility. Repeat these once or twice a day, adding each day's exercise onto the previous one/s. In addition, you should aim to take brisk aerobic exercise, ideally for at least 20 minutes per day. Use heat and ice, as explained on pages 46–47 to help prepare your joints for exercise, and to treat them afterward, if necessary. Walking and cycling are both good exercise options for the moderate program. Cycling is especially good for your hips, knees and ankles, as it flexes and extends these joints without the burden of carrying your weight. Here's a suggested regime to help you progressively increase the amount of exercise you take over the following two months. Remember to always warm up and cool down (see page 125).

- Weeks one and two: walk or cycle for 15 minutes on Tuesday, Thursday and Saturday.
- Week three: walk or cycle for 15 minutes on Thursday and for 20 minutes on Tuesday and Saturday.
- Weeks four and five: walk or cycle for 20 minutes on Tuesday, Thursday, Saturday and Sunday.
- Week six: walk or cycle for 20 minutes on Tuesday and Saturday and for 25 minutes on Thursday and Sunday.
- Week seven: walk or cycle for 25 minutes on Tuesday, Thursday, Saturday and Sunday.
- Week eight: walk or cycle for 25 minutes on Tuesday and Saturday and for 30 minutes on Thursday and Sunday.

THE MODERATE PROGRAM THERAPIES

During this program I show you some hand reflexology techniques that you can do at home followed by some techniques from other therapies. Please now book an appointment for a reflexology massage (see day seven) and to see a chiropractor (see day fourteen).

THE MODERATE PROGRAM SUPPLEMENTS

These are the supplements that I feel are most important to take on the moderate program – higher doses are suggested than for the gentle program. Read about these supplements on pages 87–93 to help you decide which you wish to take. You can, of course, take all of them, as I have designed this plan to include supplements with the best synergistic action. Supplements are widely available in pharmacies, supermarkets and healthfood stores.

Recommended daily supplements
- Chondroitin (1,200mg)
- Glucosamine sulphate (1,500mg)
- Vitamin C (1000mg)
- Omega-3 fish oils (600mg daily, for example 2 x 1g fish oil capsules, each supplying 180mg EPA + 120mg DHA)
- Evening primrose oil (1000mg)

Optional daily supplements (these provide additional benefits)
- Vitamin-B complex (50mg)
- Vitamin D (10mcg)
- Vitamin E (400iu/268mg)
- Calcium (500mg)
- Selenium (100mcg)
- Green-lipped mussel extracts (400–600mg)
- Garlic – especially if you have rheumatoid arthritis (supplying 1000mcg allicin)
- MSM (1g)

THE MODERATE PROGRAM
DAY ONE

DAILY MENU

Breakfast: Green Tea Compote (see page 180). One slice of toast
Morning snack: an apple
Lunch: Pear, Avocado and Blue Cheese Salad (see page 183). Wholemeal bread roll. Low-fat bio yogurt with black or red grapes or berries

Afternoon snack: handful of macadamias
Dinner: Pasta with Smoked Salmon and Fennel (see page 189). Green salad drizzled with Macadamia Nut and Lemon Juice Dressing (see page 186). Fresh fruit, such as plums

Drinks: 570ml/20fl oz/ scant 2⅓ cups semi-skimmed or skimmed milk. Unlimited tea (including herbal or fruit tea) and mineral water. Glass of apple juice
Supplements: see page 156

The exercises I describe over the following two weeks incorporate stretches with "range of motion" movements to help strengthen your muscles and maintain joint flexibility. Repeat these once or twice a day, adding each day's exercise to the previous ones so you build up a stretch sequence.

DAILY EXERCISE ROUTINE
Start a walking or cycling regime, as explained on page 155. Also do this simple jaw exercise.

JAW EXERCISE
1 Say your vowels by opening your mouth as wide as you can and stretching your jaw muscles in an exaggerated way:
"A … E … I … O … U".
2 Do this five times.

REFLEXOLOGY
Hand reflexology is beneficial for joints throughout your body.

HAND MASSAGE 1
1 Using an aromatherapy hand cream (for example, one that contains

> **KNOW YOUR SENSITIVITIES**
>
> You may find that certain foods in the moderate program seem to worsen your symptoms – even recognized arthritis superfoods. Avoid any foods to which you know you're sensitive (for example, acid-forming foods, see pages 79–81) and replace them with an alternative.

ginger essential oil), lightly massage between the tendons on the back of your left hand, working from your wrist to your fingers.

2 Gently massage the webbing between your fingers, and between your finger and thumb, to improve lymph circulation throughout your body, remove toxins and reduce inflammation.

3 After one or two minutes, gently squeeze the base of your thumb and slide your massaging fingers and thumb toward its tip. When you reach the base of the nail, gently squeeze the nail and slide your hand off the tip. Do this with each finger. Repeat the massage on your other hand.

DAY TWO

DAILY MENU

Breakfast: Apple, Kiwi and Watercress Smoothie (see page 180)
Morning snack: an apple
Lunch: hummus with sticks of raw carrot, celery, radish and spring onion. Foccacia bread. Low-fat bio yogurt with a handful of black or red grapes or berries
Afternoon snack: handful of Brazil nuts
Dinner: Herby Pecan Nut Roast (see page 184). Quinoa. Spinach. Carrots. Cinnamon Chocolate Nut Terrine (see page 190).

Drinks: 570ml/20fl oz/ scant 2⅓ cups semi-skimmed or skimmed milk. Unlimited tea (including herbal or fruit tea) and mineral water. Glass of apple juice
Supplements: see page 156

DAILY EXERCISE ROUTINE

Continue with your walking or cycling regime, as described on page 155. Add the following stretch to yesterday's jaw exercise.

NECK CIRCLES

1 Tilt your head to the right as if trying to rest your ear on your shoulder. Keep your shoulders relaxed and down.

2 Slowly circle your head forward so your chin is near to your chest. Keep circling it round so your left ear is as near as possible to your left shoulder. Finally, tilt your head back to complete the circle. Do five more circles.

REFLEXOLOGY

Today you're going to stimulate the solar plexus area at the top of your palm – you will find it a thumb's width below your middle finger on each side.

HAND MASSAGE 2

1 Apply pressure to the solar plexus point with your thumb and gradually push harder until you reach the limit of comfort. Hold the pressure on this reflex for at least 20 seconds, then press and release in quick pulses of one or two seconds.

2 Now gently massage across the upper palm beneath your remaining fingers, to stimulate the diaphragm line.

3 Then, as yesterday, gently squeeze the base of the thumb and slide your massaging fingers and thumb toward the tip. When you reach the base of the nail, gently squeeze the nail and slide your hand off the tip. Repeat with each finger. Now do the same with your other hand.

KNOW YOUR PAIN LIMITS

If today's neck circles hurt or make you feel dizzy, stop. The same applies to any other exercise. You should always exercise without pain, or within the limits of mild pain. If you're concerned, ask your doctor for advice on what type of exercise will suit you best.

DAY THREE

DAILY MENU

Breakfast: Fresh Figs with Blueberries (see page 180)
Morning snack: an apple
Lunch: grated beetroot (cooked or raw), carrot, courgette and Cheddar cheese arranged in four piles on a bed of mixed lettuce leaves. Brown pitta bread. Low-fat bio yogurt with a handful of black or red grapes or berries
Afternoon snack: handful of macadamia nuts
Dinner: Baked Whole Fish with Lemon and Herbs (see page 186). Wild rice. Green salad leaves drizzled with Macadamia Nut and Lemon Juice Dressing (see page 186).
Baked banana
Drinks: 570ml/20fl oz/ scant 2⅓ cups semi-skimmed or skimmed milk. Unlimited tea (including herbal or fruit tea) and mineral water. Glass of apple juice
Supplements: see page 156

To make today's dinner dessert, wrap a peeled banana in foil and bake in a moderate oven, at the same time as the fish, for 20 minutes. Serve with crème fraîche.

DAILY EXERCISE ROUTINE

Continue with your walking or cycling regime, as described on page 155. Add the following shoulder shrugs to the neck and jaw exercises of the first two days.

SHOULDER SHRUGS

1 Stand comfortably, feet apart and your arms by your sides.
2 Lift your shoulders as high as you can and keep them there for a count of three. Then relax.
3 Repeat five to 10 times.

REFLEXOLOGY

Repeat yesterday's hand massage, then I'd like you to concentrate on your spinal reflexes. These run along the outer side of your thumb, with the cervical area starting level with the base of your nail, followed by the thoracic spine, then the lumbar region in the curve where your hand and wrist meet, then the sacrum and coccyx at the side of your wrist (see diagram, page 59).

HAND MASSAGE 3

1 Gently press along the outer side of your thumb to see if you can find areas that feel gritty or tender. Focus on these by gradually pressing harder until you reach the limit of comfort.

2 Hold the pressure for at least 20 seconds, then press and release in quick pulses of one or two seconds.

3 As before, gently squeeze the base of your thumb and then slide your massaging thumb and fingers toward the top. At the base of the nail, gently squeeze and slide your fingers off the tip. Repeat with each finger. Now do the same with your other hand.

DAY FOUR

DAILY MENU

Breakfast: Omega-3 Omelette with Smoked Trout and Tarragon (see page 180)
Morning snack: an apple
Lunch: Lentil, Sweet Potato and Apricot Soup (see page 183). Wholemeal bread roll. Low-fat bio yogurt with a handful

of black or red grapes or berries
Afternoon snack: handful of Brazil nuts
Dinner: roast chicken. Braised Red Cabbage with Apple and Red Wine (see page 184). Celeriac Purée (see below). Broccoli. Fresh fruit, such as mango

Drinks: 570ml/20fl oz/ scant 2⅓ cups semi-skimmed or skimmed milk. Unlimited tea (including herbal or fruit tea) and mineral water. Glass of apple juice
Supplements: see page 156

Celeriac purée is a delicious side dish that makes an excellent alternative to potatoes. To make it, boil the celeriac for 25 minutes or until it's soft. Purée it in a food processor and then stir in some crème fraîche (or low-fat bio yogurt) and lots of black pepper. Add some nutmeg and fresh chopped parsley.

DAILY EXERCISE ROUTINE

Keep up your walking or cycling regime (see page 155). Do the stretch exercises from days one to three, then add in the following shoulder rolls.

SHOULDER ROLLS

1 Stand comfortably with your feet apart. Let both arms hang down by your sides. Slowly circle one shoulder forward, upward then backward and downward.
2 Do this five to 10 times on both shoulders, making the rolls progressively faster.

REFLEXOLOGY

Repeat yesterday's hand massage, then, after stimulating the spinal reflexes, I'd like you to move on to the sacroiliac joint reflex. This is situated on the back of each hand, just above the wrist crease and in line with your ring finger (see the diagram on page 59).

HAND MASSAGE 4

1 Gently massage the sacroiliac joint reflex. If it feels tender, increase the pressure until you reach the limit of comfort. Hold this pressure for at least 20 seconds, then press and release in quick pulses of one or two seconds.
2 As before, finish the massage by gently squeezing the base of your thumb and sliding your massaging thumb and fingers toward its top. When you reach the base of the nail, gently squeeze and slide your fingers off the tip. Repeat with each finger. Now do the same with your other hand.

DAY FIVE

Although you can't eat some of the hotter spices, such as chilli, on the moderate program, you can continue to eat black pepper (*Piper nigrum*).

This doesn't belong to the nightshade family and therefore doesn't contain glycoalkaloids that might upset your arthritis.

DAILY MENU

Breakfast: muesli (or similar high-fibre cereal with dried fruit) and semi-skimmed milk
Morning snack: an apple
Lunch: avocado and prawn open sandwich on rye bread with a scraping of olive-oil spread. Low-fat bio yogurt with black or red grapes or berries
Afternoon snack: handful of macadamia nuts
Dinner: Oaty Mackerel with Beetroot Salsa (see page 185). Mashed sweet potato. Green salad leaves drizzled with Macadamia Nut and Lemon Juice Dressing (see page 186).
Raspberry and Red Wine Sorbet (see page 190)
Drinks: 570ml/20fl oz/ scant 2⅓ cups semi-skimmed or skimmed milk. Unlimited tea (including herbal or fruit tea) and mineral water. Glass of apple juice
Supplements: see page 156

DAILY EXERCISE ROUTINE

Continue with your walking or cycling regime, as described on page 155. Do the stretches from days one to four, then add the following.

ARM BENDS

1 Tuck your hands (or just your thumbs) into your armpits. Rotate your arms so your elbows move in large circles.
2 Repeat five to 10 times.

REFLEXOLOGY

Repeat yesterday's hand reflexology massage. After stimulating the sacroiliac reflexes, move on to the hip reflexes. These are situated on the edge of each hand at the base of the little finger (see diagram on page 59).

HAND MASSAGE 5

1 Gently massage the hip reflex on your hand. If it's tender, increase the pressure up to the limit of comfort. Hold for at least 20 seconds, then press and release in quick pulses of one or two seconds.

> **SWEET POTATOES**
> Today's dinner includes mashed sweet potato (please don't substitute normal potatoes as these are members of the Solanaceae family). Sweet potato is not only more flavoursome than its regular counterpart, it's also a rich source of antioxidant carotenoids, many of which are converted into vitamin A in the body.

2 Gently squeeze the base of the thumb and slide your massaging thumb and fingers toward the top. When you reach the base of the nail, gently squeeze and then slide your hand off the tip. Repeat with each finger. Now do the same with your other hand.

DAY SIX

DAILY MENU

Breakfast: half a grapefruit (see page 120). Toast and grilled bacon **Morning snack:** an apple **Lunch:** bowl of mixed salad leaves drizzled with Macadamia Nut and Lemon Juice Dressing (see page 186). Cottage cheese with pineapple and grated beetroot. Ciabatta bread

Afternoon snack: handful of Brazil nuts **Dinner:** pasta with Pesto Sauce (see page 187). Green salad drizzled with Macadamia Nut and Lemon Juice Dressing (see page 186) and sprinkled with shavings of Parmesan cheese and mixed seeds. Berry and

Hazelnut Meringue (see page 191) **Drinks:** 570ml/20fl oz/ scant 2⅓ cups semi-skimmed or skimmed milk. Unlimited tea (including herbal or fruit tea) and mineral water. Glass of apple juice **Supplements:** see page 156

Tomorrow's lunch is going to be cold pasta and pesto salad. Prepare in advance by cooking extra pasta and pesto sauce for today's dinner and storing it in the fridge.

DAILY EXERCISE ROUTINE
Continue walking or cycling as outlined on page 155. Do the stretch exercises from days one to five, then add the following.

ARM CIRCLES

1 Raise your right arm out to your side and slowly swing it around to draw a circle in the air.

2 Do this five to 10 times, then repeat with your left arm.

REFLEXOLOGY

Repeat yesterday's hand reflexology massage, then after stimulating the hip reflexes, I'd like you to move onto the knee reflexes. These are on the edge of each hand at the base of the little finger just above the hip reflexes (see page 59).

HAND MASSAGE 6

1 Gently massage your knee reflex. If the point feels tender, increase the pressure until you reach the limit of comfort. Maintain the pressure for at least 20 seconds, then press and release in quick pulses of one or two seconds.

2 Finish the massage in the usual way: gently squeeze the base of the thumb and slide your massaging thumb and fingers toward the top. When you reach the base of the nail, gently squeeze and slide your fingers off the tip. Repeat with each finger. Now do the same with your other hand.

RED MEAT AND ARTHRITIS

Some people find that eating red meat worsens their arthritis. If your joint pains flare up over the next few days, this may be related to the bacon in today's menu. If you suspect meat brings on your symptoms, then avoid meat for the rest of this program, substituting vegetarian dishes instead (don't use tomatoes, potatoes, aubergines or bell peppers though).

DAY SEVEN

DAILY MENU

Breakfast: fruit platter: one chopped orange, one slice of watermelon, one sliced kiwi fruit, and some chopped mango. A selection of low-fat cheeses. A slice of wholegrain bread
Morning snack: an apple
Lunch: pasta with Pesto Sauce (from yesterday). Bowl of mixed green salad leaves with sprouted beans, fennel and celery, drizzled with Macadamia Nut and Lemon Juice Dressing (see page 186). Low-fat bio yogurt with a handful of black or red grapes
Afternoon snack: handful of macadamias
Dinner: Marinated Herrings (see page 186). Green salad drizzled with Macadamia Nut and Lemon Juice Dressing (see page 186). Sweetcorn. Brown rice. Fresh fruit – for example, papaya
Drinks: 570ml/20fl oz/ scant 2⅓ cups semi-skimmed or skimmed milk. Unlimited tea (including herbal or fruit tea) and mineral water. Glass of apple juice
Supplements: see page 156

DAILY EXERCISE ROUTINE

Keep up your walking or cycling routine (see page 155). Do the six exercises in your stretch sequence so far and then add today's stretch.

ARM WINDMILLS

1 Stand comfortably with your feet apart and your arms by your sides. Lift both arms forward and up, keeping them straight until they are high above your head. Then spread your arms out sideways and move them down to complete a full circle.
2 Repeat this windmill movement five to 10 times. Now do the same movements in the opposite direction five to 10 times.

CONSULTING A REFLEXOLOGIST

Having followed the moderate program for one week, you should have started to notice an improvement in your arthritis symptoms. I suggest you now visit a reflexologist. Book yourself in for four weekly sessions. Over the last week, you have learned some basic reflexology techniques that are beneficial for people with arthritis – a reflexologist will be able to show you further techniques to use. Most reflexologists work on reflexes in the feet, but some may use reflexes on your hands or ears, too. After removing your footwear, you will be asked to relax on a seat or couch with your feet raised. The therapist will lightly dust your feet with powder and will then massage your reflexes using their fingers and thumbs. Reflexologists focus on areas of tenderness and grittiness to diagnose distant problems in the body and will stimulate specific points to open up blocked nerve pathways and promote the flow of energy. A session usually lasts from 45 to 60 minutes. To find a reflexologist, check the resources on pages 235.

DAY EIGHT

DAILY MENU

Breakfast: Green Tea Compote (see page 180). One slice of wholegrain toast
Morning snack: an apple
Lunch: Tuna, Pomegranate and Anchovy Salad (see page 181). Wholemeal pitta bread. Low-fat bio yogurt with a handful of black or red grapes or berries
Afternoon snack: handful of Brazil nuts
Dinner: Pasta with Walnuts and Coriander (see page 188). Bowl of green salad leaves drizzled with Macadamia Nut and Lemon Juice Dressing (see page 186). Fresh fruit – for example, an orange
Drinks: 570ml/20fl oz/ scant 2¼ cups semi-skimmed or skimmed milk. Unlimited tea (including herbal or fruit tea) and mineral water. Glass of apple juice
Supplements: see page 156

Over the next few days I introduce several complementary therapies that can be beneficial for arthritis. Once you've found a therapy that suits you, try to find other ways to incorporate it into your daily routine.

DAILY EXERCISE ROUTINE

Continue with your walking or cycling regime, as outlined on page 155. Do the stretches you've learned so far, and then incorporate these wrist rotations.

STAYING WARM

Making sure you stay warm and avoiding cold draughts are simple but effective ways to reduce joint pain. Taking frequent hot baths or showers can also be helpful to ease joint symptoms.

WRIST CIRCLING

1 Place your palms and forearms flat on a table. Rotate your wrists so your palms turn to face upward. Try to rotate them to the point at which the backs of your hands come to rest on the table.

2 Rotate your hands back to the starting position and repeat five to 10 times.

HERBALISM

Today, I'd like you to start using a herbal medicine to help your arthritis symptoms. The remedy I've selected as most appropriate for the moderate program is ginger, which helps to suppress the release of inflammatory substances within joints. Read about it on page 42 to check that it will suit you. Start taking a ginger supplement supplying at least 300mg once or twice a day, depending on the severity of your symptoms. Choose a brand offering around 15mg gingerols (the active ingredient) per capsule.

DAY NINE

Ideally you should be taking 15 minutes of aerobic exercise three times a week. However, any exercise is better than none, so if 15 minutes is difficult, do what you can. Even pottering around the house is good for your joints.

DAILY EXERCISE ROUTINE

Keep walking or cycling (see page 155). Do the stretch exercises from days one to eight, then add the following finger-strengthening exercise.

DAILY MENU

Breakfast: Apple, Kiwi and Watercress Smoothie (see page 180)
Morning snack: an apple
Lunch: Pear, Avocado and Blue Cheese Salad (see page 183). Focaccia bread Low-fat bio yogurt with a handful of black or red grapes or berries

Afternoon snack: handful of macadamia nuts
Dinner: Baked Whole Fish with Lemon and Herbs (see page 186). Baked pumpkin, butternut squash or sweet potato. Red rice. Baked Apples with Cloves (see page 189)

Drinks: 570ml/20fl oz/ scant 2⅓ cups semi-skimmed or skimmed milk. Unlimited tea (including herbal or fruit tea) and mineral water. Glass of apple juice
Supplements: see page 156

FINGER FLEXES

1 Squeeze a soft foam ball in the palm of one hand by clenching your fingers as tightly as possible. Hold for a count of five, then relax.
2 Do this for one minute, then repeat with the other hand.

COPPER THERAPY

Today, I'd like you to buy a copper bracelet and wear it continuously for at least the remainder of this program. As described on pages 50–51, copper has the potential to reduce joint pains in people who are copper deficient.

STAY HYDRATED

Drink at least 2l (70fl oz) fluid per day to maintain good hydration and a good flow of nutrients to your joints. Choose a brand of mineral water that's rich in calcium – an important mineral for bone health. As well as water, drink fruit or herbal teas. Soup counts toward your fluid intake, too.

DAY TEN

DAILY MENU

Breakfast: porridge made with rolled oats and sprinkled with chopped banana and flaked almonds
Morning snack: an apple
Lunch: Avocado and Smoked Salmon Oriental Salad (see page 182). Wholemeal brown roll.

Low-fat bio yogurt with a handful of black or red grapes or berries
Afternoon snack: handful of Brazil nuts
Dinner: Herby Pecan Nut Roast (see page 184). Roast baby onions. Roast mushrooms. Green beans. Hemp pasta drizzled with

olive oil. Fresh fruit, for example, guava
Drinks: 570ml/20fl oz/ scant 2⅓ cups semi-skimmed or skimmed milk. Unlimited tea (including herbal or fruit tea) and mineral water. Glass of apple juice
Supplements: see page 156

DAILY EXERCISE ROUTINE

Continue to walk or cycle (see page 155). Do the nine stretch exercises you've learned so far and then add the following waist exercises.

WAIST TWISTS

1 Stand comfortably, feet slightly apart. Link your hands and stretch your arms straight out in front. Without moving your hips, swivel smoothly to the left by twisting your waist.
2 When you have twisted as far as you can, hold your position for a count of three, then return to face forward.
3 Repeat the twist to the right. Repeat the whole exercise five to 10 times.

HERBALISM

Today, I'd like you to buy a herbal preparation of arnica gel to rub into your affected joints. Apply two or three times a day for the next five days.

Note that herbal arnica gel contains between one and 25 percent *Arnica montana* extract. This contains helenalin and related compounds, which have an analgesic, anti-inflammatory action. In contrast, the homeopathic arnica gel that you may have used in the gentle program (see page 129) is prepared using the principles of homeopathy and contains no measurable amount of arnica. Make sure you choose the herbal preparation of arnica today.

LAUGHING THERAPY

Laughing is an excellent preventative measure for joint and back pains. It acts as an antidote to stress and helps you relax (stress causes clenching of muscles and tension, especially in the back area). Laughter also enhances general well-being.

DAY ELEVEN

DAILY MENU

Breakfast: Fresh Figs with Blueberries (see page 180) **Morning snack:** an apple **Lunch:** Lentil, Sweet Potato and Apricot Soup (see page 183). Wholemeal roll. Low-fat bio yogurt with a handful of black or red grapes or berries **Afternoon snack:** handful of macadamia nuts **Dinner:** Smoked Haddock Omelette with Béchamel Sauce (see page 185). Bowl of green salad leaves drizzled with Macadamia Nut and Lemon Juice Dressing (see page 186). Fresh fruit – for example, banana

Drinks: 570ml/20fl oz/ scant 2⅓ cups semi-skimmed or skimmed milk. Unlimited tea (including herbal or fruit tea) and mineral water. Glass of apple juice **Supplements:** see page 156

Macadamia nuts feature throughout the moderate program. This is because they have strong antioxidant properties that can help to reduce inflammation in the body. Macadamia nut oil has a higher percentage of monounsaturated fat than other oils – 81 percent compared to 73 percent for olive oil, 62 percent for avocado oil and 60 percent for rapeseed oil.

DAILY EXERCISE ROUTINE

Continue with your walking or cycling regime, as outlined on page 155. Do the stretches from days one to 10, then add these ankle exercises.

ANKLE ROTATIONS

1 Stand comfortably with one hand on a table for support. Lift one foot and rotate the ankle in 10 complete circles clockwise then anticlockwise.
2 Repeat with the other foot.

MAGNETIC THERAPY

Today I'd like you to apply a magnetic wrap around your most painful joint. This helps to improve circulation, warms the joint, promotes healing and reduces pain.

DAY TWELVE

DAILY MENU

Breakfast: muesli (or similar high-fibre cereal with fruit) with semi-skimmed milk
Morning snack: an apple
Lunch: Waldorf Salad (see below) on a bed of mixed green salad leaves. Ciabatta bread. Low-fat

bio yogurt with a handful of black or red grapes or berries
Afternoon snack: handful of Brazil nuts
Dinner: pork chop with rice and Delicious Black Beans (see page 187). Broccoli. Chocolate Lava

Pudding (see page 191)
Drinks: 570ml/20fl oz/ scant 2⅓ cups semi-skimmed or skimmed milk. Unlimited tea (including herbal or fruit tea) and mineral water. Glass of apple juice
Supplements: see page 156

To make the Waldorf Salad for today's lunch simply mix some chopped apple, celery and walnuts with some low-fat mayonnaise. If you're trying to lose weight, omit the ciabatta bread from your lunch and, at dinner time, eat fruit for dessert instead of Chocolate Lava Pudding. Alternatively, if you want to get the antioxidant benefits of dark chocolate without too many extra calories eat 40–50g (approximately 1½oz) by itself.

DAILY EXERCISE ROUTINE

Continue to walk or cycle (see page 155). Do the stretch exercises from days one to eleven, then add the following knee bends to your routine.

KNEE BENDS

1 Stand with your feet apart and your knees slightly bent. Put your hands on your knees. Bend your knees up and down. Don't make them completely straight and don't let your bottom go below your knees.

2 Do this five to 10 times.

HOMEOPATHY

Try one of the remedies shown in the table on page 49. Select the one that most accurately describes your arthritis symptoms. Take a 6c potency remedy twice a day for five days. Alternatively, if you consulted a homeopath after finishing the gentle program, continue with the remedies they prescribed.

MATTRESS SUPPORT

Check your mattress is not too old and saggy – ideally, you should change it every five to 10 years, depending on its quality. It's worth investing in a "memory foam" mattress if possible (see page 95).

DAY THIRTEEN

DAILY MENU

Breakfast: half a grapefruit (see caution on page 120). One slice of wholegrain toast. Mushrooms and garlic sautéed in olive oil
Morning snack: an apple
Lunch: Spicy Sweet Potato Salad (see page 182). Low-fat bio yogurt with a handful of black or red grapes or berries
Afternoon snack: handful of macadamias
Dinner: Pesto and Tuna Ciabatta Pizzas (see page 188). Green salad drizzled with Macadamia Nut and Lemon Juice Dressing (see page 186). Fresh fruit, for example, a banana
Drinks: 570ml/20fl oz/ scant 2⅓ cups semi-skimmed or skimmed milk. Unlimited tea (including herbal or fruit tea) and mineral water. Glass of apple juice
Supplements: see page 156

You can avoid stress on your hand joints by holding objects loosely and using arthritis aids such as faucet grips to help you turn taps on and off, and specially designed doorknobs that don't need to be turned or twisted. Try to hold objects in your palm rather than with your fingers, and use two hands instead of one.

DAILY EXERCISE ROUTINE

Go cycling or walking as described on page 155. Do the stretch exercises you've learned so far and then add the following heel and toe lifts.

HEEL AND TOE LIFTS

1 Start in the position you were in for yesterday's exercise (leaning forward with your hands on your knees). Lift both heels off the floor, so your calf muscles strongly contract. Lower your heels then lift your toes up toward your shins.
2 Repeat five to 10 times.

MEDITATION

Today, I'd like you to try a crystal meditation that will help you relax and will reduce pain in a particular joint. Crystals are believed to amplify the power of meditation. Choose a piece of amethyst or clear rock quartz, or another crystal that you feel particularly drawn to.

CRYSTAL MEDITATION

1 Sit comfortably in a chair with your eyes shut. Hold your crystal in both hands on your lap. Clear your mind of thoughts by focusing your attention on the crystal.
2 Visualize healing energy passing through the crystal and concentrating in your painful joint/s. Do this for 15 minutes.

DAY FOURTEEN

DAILY MENU

Breakfast: Herrings with Oatmeal and Pecan Nuts (see page 181).
Morning snack: an apple
Lunch: buffalo mozzarella and sliced mango open sandwich on rye bread with a scraping of olive-oil spread. Low-fat bio yogurt with a handful of black or red grapes or berries
Afternoon snack: handful of Brazil nuts
Dinner: risotto made with wild mushrooms (see box on page 176). Green salad drizzled with Macadamia Nut and Lemon Juice Dressing (see page 186). Fresh fruit – for example, peach
Drinks: 570ml/20fl oz/ scant 2⅓ cups semi-skimmed or skimmed milk. Unlimited tea (including herbal or fruit tea) and mineral water. Glass of apple juice
Supplements: see page 156

DAILY EXERCISE ROUTINE

Continue to walk or cycle (see page 155). Do the stretch exercises from days one to thirteen, then finish with this shaking exercise.

ARM AND LEG SHAKES

1 Shake each hand and arm in turn for a minute or two.
2 Repeat with your legs and feet. When you stop your muscles should feel soft and relaxed.

CONSULTING A CHIROPRACTOR

Having followed the moderate program for two weeks, you should have noticed a significant improvement in your arthritis; I suggest you now see a chiropractor. During a first visit, the practitioner will observe your posture and how you walk. He or she will examine your joints as you stand, sit or lie down, and you will be manoeuvred into a number of positions to assess your mobility, flexibility and nerve function. A chiropractor will use several standard neurological and orthopedic tests when assessing you, and may test your nerve reflexes and, if necessary, request x-rays. During treatment, chiropractors use their hands to help correct misalignments of the spinal vertebrae (called vertebral subluxations). The first treatment session typically lasts 30 to 60 minutes, with follow-up sessions taking 15 to 20 minutes. You may need two or three treatments during the first week followed by weekly or monthly follow-ups, although this will depend on the exact nature of your problem. To find a chiropractor, check the resources on page 234–235.

EASY RISOTTO

To make today's risotto, sauté an onion with some chopped celery and garlic in olive oil and then add 225g (8oz) wild mushrooms. Stir in 350g (12oz) risotto rice and add 150ml (5fl oz) dry white wine. Slowly add 1.2l (44fl oz) vegetable stock. When the liquid is absorbed, stir in some chopped parsley, some butter and some grated Parmesan. Season with black pepper.

CONTINUING THE MODERATE PROGRAM

Well done – you have followed the moderate program for two weeks. You now need to assess whether or not reducing your dietary exposure to nightshade plants has alleviated your arthritis symptoms. Even if you haven't noticed a significant reduction in joint pain and stiffness, I'd still like you to repeat this program so you follow it for a total of 28 days. This is because the glycoalkaloids present in members of the Solanaceae family of plants accumulate in the body, and it can take a month or so for your body to eliminate them.

YOUR LONG-TERM DIET

If, after removing nightshade glyocoalkaloids from your diet for four weeks, your symptoms have significantly improved, I suggest you continue to avoid members of the nightshade family. To help confirm the link between nightshade plants and arthritis symptoms, consider reintroducing nightshade plants for one day while monitoring your joints closely to see if your symptoms deteriorate. Symptoms produced by glycoalkaloids typically come on after eight to 12 hours, but any flare-up occurring in the one to three days after your trial reintroduction may be a result of nightshade sensitivity. If you're not certain, wait until symptoms have settled down, then reintroduce these foods again. Here's a suggested menu plan to reintroduce nightshade plants:

- Breakfast: grilled tomatoes on toast.
- Lunch: tomato soup sprinkled with paprika with one wholegrain roll.
- Dinner: Hungarian Goulash (see page 231). Mexican Hot Chilli Sauce (see page 227). Boiled, unpeeled potatoes. Tomato salad with chopped red, green and orange peppers.

If eating these foods doesn't trigger a flare-up in your symptoms, and you don't feel you have gained significant benefits from the moderate program, then either move back to the gentle program, or try the full-strength program, which offers a high intake of dietary antioxidants to help reduce joint inflammation.

If your symptoms do worsen after reintroducing nightshade plants, then you have successfully identified the link between your diet and your arthritis symptoms and you should continue to avoid eating tomatoes, potatoes, peppers, chillis, aubergines and related foods. Once you decide to stay on the moderate program long term, continue to follow the principles of the program while taking into account your own likes and dislikes. Always avoid processed, pre-packaged foods, which tend to contain high amounts of the omega-6 essential fatty acids that are converted into inflammatory substances in the body. If you do need to buy ready-foods, check the labels and avoid foods that contain ingredients such as tomatoes, potato starch, chilli, paprika and so on.

RECIPES

Explore recipes containing non-nightshade foods, especially healthy fish-based recipes. You will find some tried-and-tested recipe suggestions

REINTRODUCING POTATOES

If you want to eat a normal potato to see if you can tolerate it, make sure it's fresh, and hasn't started to turn even slightly green. Peel it thickly before cooking. Although commercial varieties of potatoes are screened for levels of the glycoalkaloid solanine, most still have a solanine content of up to 0.2mg/g. Potatoes that are exposed to light and start to turn green, however, can contain solanine concentrations of 1mg/g or more – mostly in and just under the skin. This is a natural defence to make the potato taste more bitter and therefore less likely to be eaten. Potatoes that are damaged during harvesting also produce increased levels of glycoalkaloids, as do those showing signs of disease such as blight. Eating even a single unpeeled, greening potato can result in a high dose of solanine that could make you feel quite ill and upset your joints.

at www.naturalhealthguru.co.uk and you can post your own favourites there, too, for other followers of the moderate program to try.

YOUR LONG-TERM SUPPLEMENT REGIME

Continue taking the recommended supplements long term. Research supports their use at this moderately high level for significant beneficial effects on joint health. If, up until now, you have taken only the supplements in the recommended list, you may wish to introduce one or more of the supplements in the optional list for extra benefit. Alternatively, if your arthritis symptoms are well controlled, you may wish to reduce the dose of your supplements back down to the levels suggested in the gentle program. If you feel the higher dose suits you better, you can always increase the doses back up to those suggested in the moderate program – or even increase them to those I suggest for the full-strength program.

YOUR EXERCISE ROUTINE

After doing the moderate exercises for four weeks, you should have started to notice an increase in your flexibility. Continue to do the stretch and range-of-motion exercises, ideally twice a day, and fit in the walking or cycling exercise, too (see page 155). Consider starting other activities such as swimming, dancing, gardening, bowling or golf – whatever you like doing and whatever your joints allow you to do.

You may also want to try the more advanced exercises I show you in the full-strength program – you can start incorporating those into your daily routine, too.

YOUR THERAPY PROGRAM

In the moderate program I have shown you how to use reflexology and other techniques, such as magnetic therapy, homeopathy, herbal medicine and meditation, which are beneficial for stiff, painful joints. Continue doing these, and keep going to see the natural healthcare professionals – the reflexologist and chiropractor – if you found their treatments helped relieve your symptoms.

MONITORING YOUR JOINT SYMPTOMS

Keep monitoring and scoring your joint symptoms on a weekly basis to make sure you are continuing to benefit from the moderate program. If your joint scores stop showing an improvement, or if they start to worsen again, I suggest you increase your supplement doses to those suggested for the full-strength program. Review your diet to check whether you ate any nightshade plants that might have triggered your symptoms. If not, then it's possible that you have developed a sensitivity to another food. Consult a naturopath or a nutritionist with training in the field of food intolerances. Continue to eat a balanced diet while still avoiding your individual trigger foods.

BREAKFAST RECIPES

GREEN TEA COMPOTE

SERVES 4

8 semi-dried apricots, stoned and chopped
8 semi-dried prunes, stoned and
  chopped
8 dates, stoned and chopped
8 dried figs, chopped
1 handful raisins
750ml/26fl oz/3 cups hot green tea
1 handful pistachio nuts
Low-fat fromage frais or low-fat bio
  yogurt, to serve

1 Place the fruit in a bowl, pour the
   green tea on top and leave to steep
   until cold (or overnight in the fridge).
2 Sprinkle with the pistachio nuts and
   serve with some fromage frais.

FRESH FIGS WITH BLUEBERRIES

SERVES 4

8 fresh figs
4 handfuls blueberries
125ml/4fl oz/½ cup low-fat fromage frais

1 Make two deep crosses in the tops of
   the figs, then gently open them into a
   tulip shape.
2 Mix the blueberries with the fromage
   frais, saving a few blueberries for
   garnish.
3 Put some berry mix into the figs, with
   the remainder on the side. Sprinkle
   the reserved berries over the top.

APPLE, KIWI AND WATERCRESS SMOOTHIE

SERVES 4

4 red eating apples, cored
4 kiwi fruit, peeled
1 handful of watercress
100ml/3½fl oz/scant ½ cup
  unsweetened apple juice

1 Whiz all the ingredients in a blender.

OMEGA-3 OMELETTE WITH SMOKED TROUT AND TARRAGON

SERVES 4

2 tbsp olive oil
8 omega-3-enriched eggs, lightly beaten
150g/5½oz smoked trout fillet, skinned
  and flaked
1 handful chopped tarragon
Freshly ground black pepper

1 Heat the olive oil in a large non-stick
   pan over a high heat. Tip in the eggs
   and gather the curds into the middle
   as the egg sets.
2 As soon as there's only a little runny
   egg left, remove from the heat.
   Scatter the trout and tarragon over
   one half of the omelette. Season with
   some black pepper.
3 Return to the heat and warm through
   for 30 seconds. Fold the omelette in
   half, slide out onto a plate and serve.

LUNCH RECIPES

HERRINGS WITH OATMEAL AND PECAN NUTS

SERVES 4

2 handfuls coarse oatmeal

2 handfuls pecan nuts, finely chopped

4 small herrings, cleaned, descaled with backbones removed

4 tbsp semi-skimmed milk

2 tbsp olive oil

Zest and juice of 1 unwaxed lemon

1 bunch watercress

Freshly ground black pepper

1 Mix together the oatmeal and pecans in a bowl

2 Dip the herrings in the milk and then roll them in the oatmeal mixture until evenly coated. Season with black pepper.

3 Heat the olive oil in a frying pan and fry the herrings over a gentle heat for 10 minutes on each side. Sprinkle each fish with the lemon zest and juice, and serve on a bed of watercress.

TUNA, POMEGRANATE AND ANCHOVY SALAD

SERVES 4

2 x 185g/6½oz cans tuna flakes in olive oil, drained

4 handfuls mixed salad leaves

1 handful watercress

1 bulb fennel, chopped

1 pomegranate, seeds removed (see page 142)

4 anchovy fillets in oil, drained

Ciabatta, to serve

For the dressing:

3 anchovy fillets in oil, drained

1 garlic clove, crushed

200ml/7fl oz/scant 1 cup crème fraîche

Zest and juice of 1 unwaxed lemon

Freshly ground black pepper

1 Whiz all the dressing ingredients in a blender. Season with black pepper.

2 Mix all the salad ingredients together except the anchovies and pour the dressing over the top. Sprinkle with the anchovies and serve with some ciabatta.

AVOCADO AND SMOKED SALMON ORIENTAL SALAD
SERVES 4

125g/4½oz rice noodles
1 red onion, finely chopped
½ cucumber, chopped
1 avocado, halved, stoned and peeled
100g/3½oz smoked salmon, cut in strips
1 handful mixed baby salad leaves
1 handful toasted sesame seeds

For the dressing:
4 tbsp walnut oil
1 garlic clove, crushed
1 tbsp red wine vinegar
1 tbsp chopped coriander leaves
Freshly ground black pepper

1 Cook the noodles (follow the packet instructions) and drain.

2 Put the dressing ingredients in a screw-top jar and shake well.

3 Mix all the salad ingredients together, toss them in the salad dressing and serve.

SPICY SWEET POTATO SALAD
SERVES 4

2 tbsp olive oil
1 garlic clove, crushed
1 tsp cumin seeds
1 tsp coriander seeds
2 large orange-red sweet potatoes, peeled and cubed
400g/14oz can chickpeas, drained
1 red onion, chopped
125g/4½oz/2½ cups baby spinach leaves
1 handful coriander leaves
1 handful pumpkin seeds

For the dressing:
100ml/3½fl oz/scant ½ cup low-fat bio yogurt
Zest and juice of 1 unwaxed orange
Freshly ground black pepper

1 Preheat the oven to 200°C/400°F/ Gas 6.

2 Mix the olive oil, garlic, cumin and coriander seeds in a large bowl. Toss the sweet potatoes in the spicy oil.

3 Roast the sweet potatoes for 20 minutes until tender. Mix the dressing ingredients together and season with black pepper.

4 Mix the cold sweet potatoes with the remaining salad ingredients and drizzle with the yogurt dressing.

PEAR, AVOCADO AND BLUE CHEESE SALAD

SERVES 4

2 dessert pears, quartered, cored and
   sliced
2 avocados, halved, stoned and peeled
Zest and juice of 2 unwaxed lemons
4 handfuls mixed salad leaves
100g/3½oz blue cheese (for example,
   Dolcelatte, Gorgonzola, Roquefort,
   Stilton), crumbled
55g/2oz/½ cup pecans, chopped
4 tbsp walnut oil

1 Mix the pears and avocados with the
   lemon zest and juice.

2 Put a handful of salad leaves on each
   of four plates. Pile the pear mixture
   on top and sprinkle with the blue
   cheese and the pecans. Drizzle with
   walnut oil and serve.

LENTIL, SWEET POTATO AND APRICOT SOUP

SERVES 4

2 tbsp olive oil
1 red onion, chopped
2 garlic cloves, crushed
1 tsp cumin seeds, freshly ground
3 tsp coriander seeds, freshly ground
125g/4½oz/½ cup red lentils
125g/4½oz/⅔ cup semi-dried apricots
1 sweet potato, peeled and diced
2 carrots, peeled and grated
Zest and juice of 1 unwaxed lemon
1l/35fl oz/4 cups vegetable stock
   or water
150ml/5fl oz/scant ⅔ cup low-fat
   bio yogurt
1 handful chopped coriander leaves
Freshly ground black pepper

1 Heat the olive oil in a pan and sauté
   the onion, garlic, cumin and coriander
   seeds until the onion starts to colour.
   Add all the remaining soup
   ingredients except the yogurt and
   coriander and bring to the boil.

2 Cover and simmer for 30 minutes.
   Liquidize in a blender until smooth.
   Season to taste with black pepper,
   add a swirl of yogurt and serve
   sprinkled with coriander leaves.

DINNER RECIPES

HERBY PECAN NUT ROAST

SERVES 4

1 large onion, chopped
2 garlic cloves, chopped
2 tbsp olive oil

For the herb mix:
1 handful mixed chopped herbs, for
  example, parsley, thyme, marjoram, sage
100g/3½oz/1¼ cups fresh wholemeal
  breadcrumbs
1 omega-3-enriched egg, beaten
Freshly ground black pepper

For the nut mix:
150g/5½oz/1½ cups pecan nuts, finely
  chopped
85g/3oz/1 cup fresh wholemeal
  breadcrumbs
150ml/5fl oz/scant ⅔ cup vegetable
  stock or water
Zest and juice of 1 unwaxed lemon
Freshly ground black pepper

1 Preheat the oven to 200°C/400°F/Gas 6.

2 Line a 450g/1lb loaf tin with
   non-stick, greaseproof paper. Heat
   the olive oil in a pan and sauté the
   onion and garlic. Divide the mixture
   in two. Mix one half with the herb
   mix ingredients and set aside.

3 Add the remaining onion to the nut
   mix ingredients. Put half the nut mix
   into the loaf tin. Add the herb mix,
   then the remaining nut mix.

4 Bake for 30 minutes until lightly
   brown. Allow to cool slightly, then
   turn out and serve.

BRAISED RED CABBAGE WITH APPLE AND RED WINE

SERVES 4

1 red cabbage, shredded
1 red onion, chopped
2 Red Delicious apples, cored and
  chopped
100ml/3½fl oz/scant ½ cup red wine
2 tbsp red wine vinegar
3 tbsp dark brown sugar
3 cloves
2 cinnamon sticks
¼ tsp grated nutmeg
30g/1oz butter
Freshly ground black pepper

1 Preheat the oven to 150°C/300°F/Gas 2.

2 Mix all the ingredients in a casserole
   dish. Cover and bake for 3 hours,
   stirring every half hour.

SMOKED HADDOCK OMELETTE WITH BÉCHAMEL SAUCE

SERVES 4

500ml/17fl oz/2 cups semi-skimmed milk
1 clove
1 bay leaf
1 onion, chopped
200g/7oz undyed smoked haddock,
    flaked
8 omega-3-enriched eggs, beaten
30g/1oz butter
30g/1oz/¼ cup plain flour
2 tbsp olive oil
100g/3½oz/1 cup grated Parmesan
1 handful finely chopped parsley
Freshly ground black pepper

1 Bring the milk, clove, bay leaf and
   onion to the boil in a small pan. Add
   the haddock and simmer gently until
   the fish is cooked. Remove from the
   heat.

2 Strain the milk mixture and discard
   the clove. Melt the butter in a pan
   and sprinkle the flour over the top.
   Slowly add the strained milk,
   whisking continuously until the sauce
   becomes thick and smooth.

3 Heat the olive oil in a pan and cook
   the egg until it is just set.

4 Add the flaked haddock and spoon
   over the béchamel sauce. Sprinkle
   the Parmesan over the top and and
   place under a hot grill until bubbling.
   Sprinkle with parsley, season with
   black pepper and serve.

OATY MACKEREL WITH BEETROOT SALSA

SERVES 4

4 mackerel fillets
Olive oil for brushing
1 handful rolled oats
Freshly ground black pepper

For the salsa:
2 beetroot, unpeeled
1 red onion, finely sliced
¼ cucumber, peeled and diced
2 celery sticks, finely chopped
1 carrot, peeled and grated
Zest and juice of 1 unwaxed lemon
4 tbsp extra virgin olive oil
1 handful chopped herbs, for example,
    parsley, chives, coriander

1 Preheat the oven to 200°C/400°F/Gas 6.

2 Boil the beetroot in water for 30
   minutes or until cooked. Leave to
   cool and then peel and dice.

3 Mix all the salsa ingredients and leave
   to infuse.

4 Brush the mackerel with olive oil and
   dip in the rolled oats to coat evenly.
   Season well with black pepper.

5 Put the fillets on a baking tray and
   bake for 10 minutes until cooked.
   Allow to cool and serve warm with
   the beetroot salsa.

MARINATED HERRINGS

SERVES 4

4 herring fillets, skinned and cut into
  bite-sized pieces

For the marinade:
200ml/7fl oz/scant 1 cup dry white wine
2 tbsp white wine vinegar
1 tsp clear honey
1 large spring onion, finely chopped
1 bay leaf
6 peppercorns, green, red and black
  mixed, crushed
1 handful chopped dill

For the dressing:
150ml/5fl oz/scant ⅔ cup low-fat bio
  yogurt
30g/1oz wholegrain mustard
4 tbsp chopped dill
2 tsp clear honey
Juice and zest of 1 unwaxed lemon
Freshly ground black pepper

1 Put all the marinade ingredients in a
   pan. Cover and simmer gently for 15
   minutes.

2 Put the herring fillets in a shallow dish
   and pour the boiling marinade over
   them. Cover and leave until cold.

3 Mix the dressing ingredients together
   and season to taste.

4 Remove the herring from the
   marinade (and discard the marinade).
   Mix the herring with the yogurt
   dressing and serve chilled.

MACADAMIA NUT AND LEMON JUICE DRESSING

SERVES 4

4 tbsp macadamia nut oil
Zest and juice of 1 large unwaxed lemon
Freshly ground black pepper

1 Put the ingredients in a screwtop jar
   and shake well.

BAKED WHOLE FISH WITH LEMON AND HERBS

SERVES 4

1.5kg/3lb 5oz whole round fish (for
  example, sea bass, grey mullet, trout,
  salmon), boned, gutted, descaled and
  washed
2 tbsp olive oil (or herb-flavoured olive
  oil)
1 handful mixed herbs, for example,
  fennel, dill, thyme, rosemary
1 handful chopped parsley
1 unwaxed lemon, sliced
Freshly ground black pepper

1 Preheat the oven to 190°C/375°F/Gas 5.

2 Brush the fish inside and out with the
   olive oil and season with black
   pepper. Fill the body of the fish with
   the herbs and put the lemon slices on
   the outside of the fish.

3 Wrap the fish in foil and bake for
   30–45 minutes until it is cooked
   through.

DELICIOUS BLACK BEANS

SERVES 4

2 tbsp olive oil

1 large onion, chopped

2 garlic cloves, crushed

2 celery sticks, finely chopped

1 large carrot, peeled and grated

1 handful chopped mixed herbs, for
   example, parsley, oregano, basil

1 pinch ground cloves

225g/8oz dried black beans, washed and
   soaked overnight (keep the liquid)

1 stock cube (beef, chicken or vegetable)

1 bay leaf

2 tsp red wine vinegar

Freshly ground black pepper

1 Heat the olive oil in a pan and sauté
   the onion, garlic, celery, carrot, herbs
   and ground cloves until the onion
   starts to brown.

2 Add the beans to the onion mixture
   together with some of the soaking
   liquid – enough to cover the
   ingredients by at least 5cm/2in.

3 Add the stock cube and bay leaf and
   bring to the boil. Cover and simmer
   for 2 hours, stirring occasionally. Stir
   in the vinegar and season well with
   black pepper. Continue cooking for a
   further 30 minutes. Remove the bay
   leaf and serve.

PESTO SAUCE

SERVES 4

55g/2oz/1 cup firmly packed basil leaves

55g/2oz/½ cup pecan nuts, chopped

3 garlic cloves, crushed

185ml/6fl oz/¾ cup extra virgin olive oil

1 handful freshly grated Parmesan
   cheese

1 handful freshly grated pecorino cheese
   (or more Parmesan)

Freshly ground black pepper

1 Whiz all the ingredients in a blender
   until smooth. Or, if you prefer a
   coarser texture, grind each ingredient
   in turn using a pestle and mortar,
   then add the olive oil a little at a time.

2 Season with black pepper to taste.

PESTO AND TUNA CIABATTA PIZZAS

SERVES 4

2 part-baked ciabatta, halved
lengthways
1 recipe quantity Pesto Sauce
(see previous recipe)
185g/6½oz can flaked tuna in olive oil,
drained
1 handful black olives, pitted and halved
4 handfuls grated cheese (Cheddar or
mozzarella)
Freshly ground black pepper

1 Preheat the oven to 180°C/350°F/Gas 4.

2 Spread each half of the ciabattas with
pesto and place cut-side up on a
baking sheet. Sprinkle each one with
a quarter of the flaked tuna, olives
and cheese. Bake for 20 minutes.

PASTA WITH WALNUTS AND CORIANDER

SERVES 4

6 tbsp walnut oil
4 handfuls walnuts, chopped
2 garlic cloves, crushed
1 tsp coriander seeds, crushed
1 handful chopped coriander leaves
450g/1lb fresh pasta or 350g/12oz
dried pasta
60g/2oz/⅔ cup grated Parmesan
Freshly ground black pepper

1 Blend or pound the walnut oil,
walnuts, garlic, coriander seeds and
leaves into a smooth paste. Season
with black pepper.

2 Cook the pasta in plenty of boiling
water until al dente. Drain but leave
moist so the sauce will coat the
pasta well.

3 Mix the pasta with the walnut and
coriander mixture, toss well and
sprinkle with Parmesan. Leave to
marinate for at least 1 hour, then
reheat and serve.

DESSERT RECIPES

PASTA WITH SMOKED SALMON AND FENNEL
SERVES 4

2 tbsp olive oil
2 garlic cloves, crushed
1 onion, chopped
1 small bulb fennel, chopped into matchsticks (reserve the green fronds)
Zest and juice of 1 unwaxed lemon
300ml/10½fl oz/1¼ cups Greek yogurt
200g/7oz smoked salmon, chopped
450g/1lb fresh wholemeal pasta or 350g/12oz dried pasta
Freshly ground black pepper

1 Heat the olive oil in a pan and sauté the garlic, onion and chopped fennel until starting to colour. Add the lemon zest and juice, and yogurt. Heat through, stirring continuously. Don't boil or the yogurt may curdle.

2 Remove from the heat and stir in the smoked salmon. Meanwhile, cook the pasta in plenty of boiling water until al dente. Drain but leave moist so the sauce will coat the pasta well. Combine the pasta and sauce. Season with some black pepper.

3 Toss well, sprinkle the chopped fennel fronds on top and serve.

BAKED APPLES WITH CLOVES
SERVES 4

55g/2oz/⅓ cup semi-dried apricots, chopped
750ml/26fl oz/3 cups hot tea (black, green or white)
4 cooking apples, cored
16 cloves
55g/2oz/½ cup raisins
55g/2oz butter
55g/2oz/¼ cup firmly packed soft brown sugar

1 Preheat the oven to 180°C/350°F/Gas 4.

2 Soak the apricots in hot tea for 10 minutes. Meanwhile, peel the top quarter of each apple and stud the flesh with 4 cloves. Place in a baking dish.

3 Mix the soaked apricots with the raisins, butter and sugar. Use the mixture to fill the cored centre of each apple. Pour a little hot tea in the dish with the apples to a depth of around 3mm/⅛in.

4 Bake for 45 minutes until the apples are soft. Remove the cloves and serve with the juice from the pan.

RASPBERRY AND RED WINE SORBET

SERVES 4

250g/9oz/2 cups raspberries, fresh or
    thawed from frozen
200ml/7fl oz/scant 1 cup light red wine,
    for example, Beaujolais, Valpolicella
55g/2oz/¼ cup granulated sugar

1 Put all the ingredients in a pan and
   bring to the boil, stirring until the
   sugar dissolves. Simmer for 5 minutes.
2 Cool and put in the freezer for 3
   hours, churning up the ice crystals
   occasionally.

CINNAMON CHOCOLATE NUT TERRINE

SERVES 8

Oil, for brushing
400g/14oz dark chocolate (at least
    70 percent cocoa solids)
300ml/10½fl oz/scant 1¼ cup double
    cream
2 tsp ground cinnamon
1 tbsp caster sugar
350g/12oz/3½ cups pecan nuts, halved

1 Lightly brush a 20cm x 13cm (8in x 5in)
   loaf tin with the oil, and line with
   clingfilm – leave some overhanging.
   Partially melt the chocolate on a plate
   over hot water. Heat the cream to
   just below boiling point.
2 Remove the partially melted
   chocolate from the heat and add
   the hot cream, stirring well, until
   the chocolate fully melts.
3 Stir in the cinnamon and caster sugar.
   Place a layer of pecan nuts in the
   bottom of the loaf tin, and pour over
   some of the chocolate mixture. Keep
   layering, finishing with chocolate. Chill
   for 2 hours, then remove from the tin,
   discard the clingfilm and serve.

CHOCOLATE LAVA PUDDING
SERVES 6

100g/3½oz soft, unsalted butter
  (keep the butter paper)
55g/2oz/½ cup plain flour (plus extra
  for dusting)
300g/10½oz dark chocolate (at least
  70 percent cocoa solids)
125g/4½oz/⅔ cup golden caster sugar
4 omega-3-enriched eggs, beaten
1 tsp vanilla extract

1 Preheat the oven to 200°C/400°F/
  Gas 6.

2 Use the butter paper to grease 6
  ramekins. Then dust with flour. Melt
  the chocolate on a plate over hot
  water.

3 Cream together the butter and sugar,
  then beat in the eggs and vanilla
  extract. Add the flour to make a
  smooth batter, then mix in the
  chocolate.

4 Divide the mixture between the
  ramekins and cook for 10 minutes.
  Serve hot.

BERRY AND HAZELNUT MERINGUE
SERVES 4

4 omega-3-enriched eggs, whites only
200g/7oz/¾ cup plus 1 tbsp caster
  sugar
250ml/9fl oz vanilla/1 cup low-fat
  fromage frais
300g/10½oz berries, for example,
  strawberries, raspberries, blueberries
  or blackberries
100g/3½oz/¾ cup toasted hazelnuts,
  chopped
1 small handful chopped mint leaves

1 Preheat the oven to 140°C/275°F/Gas 1.

2 Beat the egg whites until they form
  stiff peaks. Gradually beat in the
  sugar to form a glossy, thick, white
  meringue. Spread the meringue in a
  circle (roughly 23cm/9in in diameter)
  on a sheet of non-stick baking
  parchment.

3 Bake in the oven for around 1 hour,
  or until the meringue is crisp on the
  outside. Remove and allow to cool.

4 Spread the fromage frais over the
  meringue and sprinkle the berries,
  toasted hazelnuts and mint on top.

INTRODUCING THE FULL-STRENGTH PROGRAM

The full-strength program is ideal for people whose arthritis symptoms didn't significantly improve while following the Mediterranean-style diet of the gentle program or the exclusion diet of the moderate program. I also recommend it if your arthritis is associated with the inflammation (red, swollen joints) that's common in rheumatoid and other autoimmune forms of arthritis.

THE FULL-STRENGTH PROGRAM DIET

The full-strength program offers a way to eat that is exceptionally high in antioxidants. It incorporates foods with a high Oxygen Radical Absorbance Capacity (ORAC; see pages 72–75) value, such as dark chocolate, blueberries, red kidney beans, cranberries, Red Delicious apples, Russet potatoes and plums – these typically provide more than 4,000 ORAC units per average serving. Some of the other arthritis superfoods in the program offer fewer ORAC units, but I've made sure that they each provide more than 1,000 ORAC units per average serving – they soon add up.

The average person eating a typical Western diet obtains an estimated 5,700 ORAC units a day. Ideally, you need to obtain at least 7,000 ORAC units a day for good health. The full-strength program offers you at least 20,000 ORAC units per day from diet alone. This has the potential to significantly reduce inflammation linked to free-radical damage within your joints.

EATING LOTS OF CHILLIES

The full-strength program diet includes chillies and other spices, which, as well as having an antioxidant potential, also have a medicinal, analgesic action in the body. Chilli peppers contain natural analgesic compounds known as capsaicinoids and are particularly beneficial for arthritis – as long as you're not sensitive to the nightshade family of plants (see pages 77–78). As the full-strength program also includes other members of the nightshade family – potatoes, tomatoes, peppers and aubergines – you

SHOPPING LIST

Base your shopping lists on the following items, which feature in the menu plans and recipes. Buy regularly in small quantities.

DRINKS

apple juice (unsweetened), blueberry juice, cranberry juice, fruit teas, green, black or white tea, herbal teas, mineral water (low sodium), pomegranate juice, red wine (Beaujolais)

DAIRY PRODUCTS

butter (unsalted), crème fraîche, fromage frais (plain and vanilla), semi-skimmed or skimmed cows' milk, vanilla ice-cream (low fat), yogurt (plain low-fat bio); cheeses: cottage cheese, Cheddar, feta, Gruyère, mozzarella, Parmesan,

FRUIT

apples (Red Delicious and cooking apples), bananas, blackberries, blueberries, cherries, cranberries (dried and fresh), dates, figs (dried and fresh), grapes (black), kiwi fruit, lemons, limes, mangoes, oranges, peaches, plums, prunes, raisins, raspberries, strawberries

VEGETABLES

aubergines, avocados, beetroot, black beans, broccoli, cabbage (red), carrots, celery, chickpeas, courgettes, cucumber, florence fennel, globe artichoke, green beans, kale, kidney beans (dried), lentils (red), lettuce (red oak leaf, lollo rosso, little gem), mixed red salad leaves, onions (red), peas, purple sprouting broccoli, red kidney beans, Russet potatoes, spinach, sweetcorn, bell peppers (red, green, yellow), sweet potatoes, tomatoes (regular and beef)

NUTS AND SEEDS

almonds, mixed seeds, pecans, pistachios, walnuts

HERBS, SPICES, OILS AND VINEGAR

basil, bay leaf, black pepper (freshly ground), cardamom pods, chillies (red, green), chilli powder, cinnamon (ground and sticks), cloves (whole), coriander (powder, leaves and seeds), cumin, dill, fenugreek, garlic, ginger, mustard seeds, oregano/marjoram, paprika (hot), paprika (sweet), parsley, peppercorns (black, pink), saffron stamens, turmeric; extra virgin and standard olive oil, pecan nut oil, walnut oil; red wine vinegar, rice wine vinegar

GRAINS

bulgur wheat, high-fibre breakfast cereals, noodles, porridge oats, rice (Basmati, brown, long grain and red), speciality breads (ciabatta, focaccia, garlic and herb, sun-dried tomato), wholegrain/multigrain bread and rolls, wholemeal flour (plain, self-raising), wholemeal pitta bread

PROTEINS

omega-3-enriched eggs; fish: mackerel (smoked), prawns, salmon (fresh and smoked), tuna (fresh or in olive oil), white fish (for example, bream, red snapper or sea bass); meat: beef (lean fillet), chicken fillet, ham, stewing steak

MISCELLANEOUS

baking powder, bean salad (tinned), black bean sauce (organic), coconut milk, desiccated coconut, dark chocolate (at least 70 percent cocoa solids), dried skimmed milk powder, gelatine powder, honey (runny), maple syrup, mayonnaise (low fat), mustard (wholegrain), olive-oil spread, red pesto sauce, tomato purée, stock cubes (vegetable), sugar (Demerara, golden caster, icing and white), tortilla chips, vanilla pod or extract, vanilla essence need to be sure that eating them doesn't worsen your arthritis. If you're unsure, go back and complete the moderate program to find out.

Capsaicinoids (examples include capsaicin, dihydrocapsaicin, nordihydrocapsaicin, homodihydrocapsaicin and homocapsaicin), are irritants found in the flesh of chilli peppers – they are especially concentrated in the white tissue supporting the seeds. As well as producing the burning sensations that occur when you eat chillies, capsaicinoids have painkilling properties. They overwhelm pain-detecting nerves and prevent them from passing on further pain messages. Capsaicin also blocks the activity of decapeptide substance P (DSP), thereby protecting against cartilage breakdown in osteoarthritis.

The capsaicin content and hotness of chilli peppers is measured according to the Scoville scale (see page 214), in which a sweet bell pepper has a Scoville rating of zero (no capsaicin) while the hottest chilli, the habanero, has a rating of 200,000 plus – meaning that its juice must be diluted more than 200,000 times before the capsaicin becomes undetectable. The hotter the pepper, the higher the capsaicin content and the more potentially beneficial it is for arthritis pain.

EATING OTHER ARTHRITIS SUPERFOODS

The full-strength diet features red lentils, which are one of the richest plant sources of protein and which also have an unusually high ORAC score. It also includes beetroot – a source of unique pigments called betalains (for example, betanin) which, as well as giving beetroot its dark, attractive colour and earthy flavour, have a powerful antioxidant action.

For your daily snacks, I have suggested high-ORAC-score fruits, such as berries and Red Delicious apples. During this program, your daily nut snack consists of either pecans or walnuts, which, as well as having an excellent antioxidant content, are good sources of anti-inflammatory, omega-3 fatty acids.

LOSING WEIGHT

Although it's not designed for weight loss, you should find that you lose any excess weight slowly and naturally while following this healthy-eating

FULL-STRENGTH PROGRAM SUPPLEMENTS

These are the supplements that I feel are the most beneficial on the full-strength program. Read about them on pages 87–93 to help you decide which you wish to take. You can, of course, take all of them, as I have designed this plan to include supplements with the best synergistic action. Supplements are widely available from pharmacies, supermarkets and healthfood stores.

Recommended daily supplements

- Glucosamine sulphate (1,500mg)
- Chondroitin (1,200mcg)
- MSM (1g)
- Vitamin C (1000mg, twice daily)
- Omega-3 fish oils (900mg daily, for example, 3 x 1g fish oil capsules, each supplying 180mg EPA + 120mg DHA)
- Evening primrose oil (2,000mg)

Optional daily supplements (these provide additional benefits)

- Vitamin-B complex (75mg)
- Vitamin D (15mcg)
- Vitamin E (400mg/600i.u.)
- Calcium (800mg)
- Selenium (200mcg)
- Green-lipped mussel extracts – especially for inflammatory forms of arthritis such as rheumatoid (600–900mg)
- Garlic tablets – especially if you have rheumatoid arthritis (allicin yield 1,500 mcg)

program. If you want to speed up the process of weight loss, eat smaller portions, especially of the starchy foods such as pasta, bread and rice – and replace dessert recipes with high-ORAC fruits.

THE FULL-STRENGTH PROGRAM EXERCISE ROUTINE

Your exercise routine involves a series of stretches that have been designed to improve your joint flexibility. Repeat these once or twice a day, adding each day's exercise to the previous one/s. In addition, you should aim to take regular brisk aerobic exercise. Use heat and ice, as explained on page 46–47, to help prepare your joints for exercise, and to treat them afterward if necessary.

Walking, cycling and swimming are all good choices of aerobic exercise. Swimming helps to build strength, stamina and suppleness and is especially good for weight-bearing joints, such as your back, hips, knees and ankles. Here's a suggested regime to follow to help you slowly increase the amount of exercise you take over the full-strength program (plus the month after), whether you select walking, cycling or swimming. Remember to warm up and cool down first.

- Week one: walk, cycle or swim for 20 minutes on Tuesday, Thursday and Saturday.
- Week two: walk, cycle or swim for 20 minutes on Tuesday and Saturday, and for 25 minutes on Thursday.
- Week three: walk, cycle or swim for 20 minutes on Thursday and Sunday, and for 25 minutes on Tuesday and Saturday.
- Week four: walk, cycle or swim for 25 minutes on Tuesday, Thursday, Saturday and Sunday.
- Week five: walk, cycle or swim for 25 minutes on Thursday and Sunday, and for 30 minutes on Tuesday and Saturday.
- Week six: walk, cycle or swim for 30 minutes on Tuesday, Thursday, Saturday and Sunday.
- Week seven: walk, cycle or swim for 30 minutes on Thursday and Sunday, and for 35 minutes on Tuesday and Saturday.
- Week eight: walk, cycle or swim for 35 minutes on Tuesday and Saturday, and for 40 minutes on Thursday and Sunday.

THE FULL-STRENGTH PROGRAM THERAPIES

During this program, I show you some acupressure techniques to do at home, followed by other holistic approaches. I suggest that you book an appointment with an acupuncturist and a Reiki practitioner now in preparation for days seven and fourteen.

THE FULL-STRENGTH PROGRAM
DAY ONE

DAILY MENU

Breakfast: toast with Berry and Apple Jelly (see page 222)
Morning snack: Red Delicious apple or a handful of black grapes
Lunch: globe artichoke with chopped dates, figs, tomatoes, basil and mozzarella cheese. Mixed red salad leaves drizzled with Pecan Nut Oil and Red Wine Vinegar

Dressing (see page 225). Pitta bread. "High-ORAC" fruit (see pages 74–75)
Afternoon snack: handful of pecans
Dinner: Extra-spicy Chilli Beans (see page 231). Red rice. Mashed avocado with lemon juice. Mixed red salad leaves drizzled with Pecan Nut Oil and Red Wine Vinegar Dressing (see page 225).

40–50g (about 1½oz) bar dark chocolate. A handful of cherries
Drinks: 570ml/20fl oz/ scant 2⅓ cups semi-skimmed or skimmed milk. Unlimited tea (including herbal or fruit tea) and mineral water. Glass of pomegranate, blueberry, cranberry or apple juice
Supplements: see page 195

Your dinner tonight is extra-spicy chilli beans. If you have a good tolerance for spicy food, add some Mexican hot chilli sauce – the analgesic compounds in chillies are good for your joints.

DAILY EXERCISE ROUTINE

The exercises I show you over the following two weeks are stretches that will help strengthen your muscles and maintain your joint flexibility. They will help you to stay active and mobile. Repeat them once or twice a day, adding each day's exercise to the ones you've learned previously. You should also start your walking, cycling or swimming regime, as described on pages 195–196.

FORWARD STRETCHES

1 Stand comfortably, feet slightly apart, arms by your sides. Bend forward as if to touch your toes.
2 Stretch down with your arms and fingers as far down your legs as is comfortable.
3 Maintain your maximum stretch for five seconds. Flex your knees

slightly and put your hands on your knees to help you stand up. Stand straight with your shoulders back and relax before repeating the stretch at least once more.

ACUPRESSURE

During the first week of the program, I'm going to show you how to use acupressure to reduce joint pain. Today's acupressure point is Large Intestine 4, also known as LI4, *HeGu* or Union Valley – don't use this point if you are pregnant.

LARGE INTESTINE 4

1 LI4 is on the back of your hand in the web between your thumb and index finger. To find it, bring your thumb and index finger close together and feel around the highest spot of the muscle bulge that forms from the web on the back of your hand – it is likely to feel tender. Press lightly, and gradually increase the pressure to the limit of comfort.
2 Release the pressure gradually and then build it up. Press for one minute while breathing slowly and deeply. If your joint pains are worse on your left side, use LI4 on your right hand for relief, and vice versa.

DAY TWO

DAILY MENU

Breakfast: Apple and Carrot Breakfast Muffins (see page 221)
Morning snack: Red Delicious apple or a handful of black grapes
Lunch: Borscht Soup (see page 224). Wholegrain roll. "High-ORAC" fruit (see page 74–75)

Afternoon snack: handful of walnuts
Dinner: poached or steamed fish fillet. Spinach. Carrots drizzled with low-fat bio yogurt. Mashed Russet potatoes. Chocolate, Prune and Pecan Squares (see page 233)

Drinks: 570ml/20fl oz/ scant 2⅓ cups semi-skimmed or skimmed milk. Unlimited tea (including herbal or fruit tea) and mineral water. Glass of pomegranate, blueberry, cranberry or apple juice
Supplements: see page 195

DAILY EXERCISE ROUTINE

Continue with the walking, cycling or swimming regime suggested on pages 195–196. Do yesterday's forward stretch, then these side bends. If today's exercise, or any other exercise, makes you feel dizzy, unstable or uncomfortable, stop straightaway – see the caution about knowing your limits on page 159.

SIDE BENDS

1 Stand comfortably with your feet apart and your hands by your sides. Slowly bend sideways to your left, so your left hand travels down your leg as far as is comfortable.
2 Slowly straighten and repeat on the right side. (Take care not to lean forward or backward as you bend.) Repeat so that you do five bends to the left and five to the right.
3 To make this exercise easier, flex your knees slightly and walk your hands up your legs when you stand up from a bend. You can also stabilize yourself by doing the exercise with your back against a wall.

ACUPRESSURE

Work on yesterday's acupressure point and then today's: Governing Vessel 14, also known as DU14, *DaZhui* or the Great Hammer. This point is used in Chinese medicine to strengthen the neck and spine, and to dispel the invasion of wind and cold that in Chinese medicine is believed to be responsible for causing painful muscles and joints.

GOVERNING VESSEL 14

1 This point is located between your seventh cervical (neck) vertebra and the spinous process of your first thoracic vertebra, approximately level with your shoulders. To find it, bend your head forward and run a finger down the back of your neck. Find the most prominent bone and then feel for the hollow just beneath – it may feel slightly tender.
2 Stimulate the point by slowly increasing the pressure to the limit of comfort and then gradually releasing it. Keep pressing in this way for one minute while breathing slowly and deeply.

DAY THREE

DAILY MENU

Breakfast: Omelette with Caramelized Sweet Potato and Red Onions (see page 222). Wilted baby spinach. Sliced tomatoes

Morning snack: Red Delicious apple or a handful of black grapes

Lunch: smoked mackerel. Shredded red cabbage, carrot, beetroot and red onion. Mixed red salad leaves with Pecan Nut Oil and Red Wine Vinegar Dressing (see page 225). Speciality bread. "High-ORAC" fruit (see pages 74–75)

Afternoon snack: handful of pecans

Dinner: Hungarian Goulash (see page 231). Red or brown rice. Mixed red salad leaves with Pecan Nut Oil and Red Wine Vinegar Dressing (see page 225). Vanilla ice cream with Fresh Strawberry Coulis (see page 232)

Drinks: 570ml/20fl oz/ scant 2⅓ cups semi-skimmed or skimmed milk. Unlimited tea (including herbal or fruit tea) and mineral water. Glass of pomegranate, blueberry, cranberry or apple juice

Supplements: see page 195

DAILY EXERCISE ROUTINE

Walk, cycle or swim (see pages 195–196) and do the stretch exercises from days one and two, followed by these wall presses.

WALL PRESSES

1 Stand facing a wall with your feet hip-width apart, your back straight, your abdominal muscles pulled in and your pelvis tilted forward. Place your hands flat on the wall in line with your shoulders.
2 Bend your elbows and lean in so your nose almost touches the wall – keep your back flat and your legs straight. Hold this position briefly then use your arms to push away from the wall. Breathe in as you lean in; breathe out as you push out. Repeat five to 10 times.

ACUPRESSURE

Work on the sequence of acupressure points you have learned so far, then stimulate Bladder 11, also known as Bl11, *DaShu* or Great Shuttle point. This will disperse wind from your joints and bones.

BLADDER 11

1 Locate the point two finger widths away from the spine on either side – below the Great Hammer (see page 199), level with the space between your first and second thoracic vertebrae.

2 Stimulate Bl11 on your left side by putting your right hand over your left shoulder, and vice versa. Stimulate as usual by slowly increasing pressure then releasing it over a period of a minute while breathing slowly and deeply.

RED WINE

Feel free to drink red wine (but stick to two or three glasses a week). The antioxidant activity of one glass (150ml/5fl oz) of red wine is equivalent to that of 12 glasses of white wine. Watch out for any flare-up in your arthritis symptoms a day or two after drinking wine though – some people have an alcohol intolerance.

DAY FOUR

DAILY MENU

Breakfast: Cinnamon Toast (see page 221). Chopped banana **Morning snack:** Red Delicious apple or a handful of black grapes **Lunch:** Potato Salad (see page 202). Cottage cheese with dates and pistachios. Bowl of mixed red salad leaves with Pecan Nut Oil and Red Wine Vinegar Dressing (see page 225).

"High-ORAC" fruit (see pages 74–75) **Afternoon snack:** handful of walnuts **Dinner:** grilled aubergine, red, green and yellow peppers, red onion, and courgette, brushed with olive oil and sprinkled with Mexican Hot Chilli Sauce (see page 227). Red Lentil Dhal (see page 228). Mashed sweet potato. Purple sprouting broccoli.

40–50g (about 1½oz) bar dark chocolate and/or a handful of raspberries **Drinks:** 570ml/20fl oz/ scant 2⅓ cups semi-skimmed or skimmed milk. Unlimited tea (including herbal or fruit tea) and mineral water. Glass of pomegranate, blueberry, cranberry or apple juice **Supplements:** see page 195

To make the potato salad at lunchtime, boil chopped Russet potatoes with the skins on. Leave them to cool, then mix them with chopped red onion and low-fat mayonnaise.

When you grill the red peppers and cook the red lentil dhal for dinner, make extra for tomorrow's lunch.

DAILY EXERCISE ROUTINE
Go for a walk, cycle or swim (see pages 195–196). Do the stretch exercises from days one to three, then add the following leg stretch.

LEG STRETCH
1 Stand with your left side near a wall, your left hand on the wall.
2 Bend your left knee slightly, then bend your right leg behind you and grasp your right ankle with your right hand. Keep your knees facing forward (don't twist them). Ease your foot toward your bottom. Hold for a count of five. Turn round, and repeat on the other side.

ACUPRESSURE
Stimulate the acupoints from previous days, then work on Stomach 36, also known as St36, *ZuSanLi* or Leg Three Miles.

STOMACH 36
1 Locate the point four fingerwidths below your kneecap to the outside of the shinbone in a hollow that forms when you bend your knee, between the shin bone and the leg muscle.

THE RIGHT WALKING STICK
If you use a walking stick, select one with a T-shaped handle, which offers better support than a crook-shape. Check it's the correct height by standing up straight with your usual walking shoes on and your arms at your sides. The top of the stick should reach the crease on the underside of your wrist. This allows your elbow to flex to 15 to 20 degrees when you hold the stick while standing.

2 Gradually build up the pressure on the acupoint and then gradually release it. Do this for about one minute, while breathing slowly and deeply. Now repeat on the other leg.

DAY FIVE

DAILY MENU

Breakfast: Apple and Raspberry Smoothie (see page 223) **Morning snack:** Red Delicious apple or a handful of black grapes **Lunch:** Kidney Bean, Beetroot and Feta Salad (see page 224). Cold grilled red pepper drizzled with olive oil. Cold red lentil dhal. Wholegrain roll (optional). "High-ORAC" fruit (see pages 74–75) **Afternoon snack:** handful of pecans **Dinner:** Mango Salsa Salmon Steaks (see page 230). Broccoli. Green peas. Baked Russet potato. Baked or stewed apple with vanilla fromage frais **Drinks:** 570ml/20fl oz/ scant 2⅓ cups semi-skimmed or skimmed milk. Unlimited tea (including herbal or fruit tea) and mineral water. Glass of pomegranate, blueberry, cranberry or apple juice **Supplements:** see page 195

Make a pot of green tea this evening and put some prunes in the liquid while still hot. Leave the prunes to soak overnight, so that they're ready for tomorrow's breakfast.

DAILY EXERCISE ROUTINE

Walk, swim or cycle (see pages 195–196). Do the first four exercises of the program followed by the wall sits below.

WALL SITS

1 Stand with your back a little way away from a wall, your feet hip-width apart and your toes pointing forward. Lean back and press your lower back into the wall. Pull in your abdominals, relax your shoulders, and bend your knees and hips to around 90 degrees.
2 Hold this position for as long as is comfortable – at least 10 seconds at first, building up to one minute eventually.

ACUPRESSURE

Today's point is used specifically to treat arthritis of the knee joint. It's called Stomach 35, St35, *DuBi* or Calf's Nose. Stimulate this point after you've worked on the acupoints on days one to four.

STOMACH 35

1 This point is located just below the knee. To find it, bend your knee and search with your fingers in the outside dimple of your knee joint, below the kneecap on the outside of the ligament.
1 Press lightly, then slowly increase the pressure to the limit of comfort. Release the pressure gradually and build it up again to stimulate the point. Continue pressing for about one minute, while breathing slowly and deeply. Repeat on the other side.

DAY SIX

DAILY MENU

Breakfast: prunes soaked overnight in green tea, sprinkled with pistachios
Morning snack: Red Delicious apple or a handful of black grapes
Lunch: slice of ham, cheese or smoked salmon. Spiced Lentil Salad (see page 226). Mixed red salad leaves with Pecan Nut Oil and Red Wine Vinegar

Dressing (see page 225). "High-ORAC" fruit (see pages 74–75)
Afternoon snack: handful of walnuts
Dinner: grilled chicken fillet marinated in olive oil, garlic and herbs. Green beans. Saffron Rice (see page 229). Blueberry and Cranberry Jelly (see page 233)

Drinks: 570ml/20fl oz/ scant 2⅓ cups semi-skimmed or skimmed milk. Unlimited tea (including herbal or fruit tea) and mineral water. Glass of pomegranate, blueberry, cranberry or apple juice
Supplements: see page 195

Today you will be discovering the last acupressure point in the sequence of six. From today, check the acupressure points you've used during the full-strength program on a daily basis. Continue to massage those that are still tender.

DAILY EXERCISE ROUTINE

Continue to walk, cycle or swim, as outlined on pages 195–196. Do the stretches from the previous days, then add these mini squats.

MINI SQUATS

1 Stand with your hands on your hips, your feet 1m (approx 3ft) apart, and your toes turned out. Bend your knees, and, keeping your knees turned out over your toes, squat down as low as you can – taking care not to lean forward.

1 Lift up and down using slow movements. Do this 10 times initially, and work up to 20.

ACUPRESSURE

The final acupressure point I'd like to introduce to you is Triple Heater 6, also known as SJ6, *ZhiGou* or Branch Ditch. It's used to dispel stagnant qi in the upper body, and to treat shoulder and back pain.

TRIPLE HEATER 6

1 You can find this point four finger widths above your wrist on the back of your forearm, between your two lower arm bones.

2 Press lightly on this point, and gradually increase the pressure as much as you can tolerate. Release the pressure gradually and build it up again to stimulate the point. Continue this for about one minute, while breathing slowly and deeply. Repeat on the other side.

SITTING COMFORTABLY

If you can, invest in an adjustable chair – it will support your back and help prevent pain. When sitting, move your hips back as far as you can until they are against the back of the chair. Then, adjust the seat height until your feet are flat on the floor. Your hips should be at the same height or slightly higher than your knees. Adjust the backrest, if possible, so that it is comfortably resting in the curve of your lower back.

DAY SEVEN

DAILY MENU

Breakfast: Apple, Kiwi and Blueberry Smoothie (see page 223)
Morning snack: Red Delicious apple or a handful of black grapes
Lunch: Salmon and Mixed Bean Lunch Bowl (see page 225). Speciality bread, such as sun-dried tomato bread or garlic and herb bread.

"High-ORAC" fruit (see page 74–75)
Afternoon snack: handful of pecans
Dinner: Extra-spicy Chilli Beans (see page 231). Tortilla chips. Mashed avocado (mixed with lemon or lime juice and crème fraîche). Mexican Hot Chilli Sauce (see page 227). Chocolate, Prune

and Pecan Squares (see page 233)
Drinks: 570ml/20fl oz/ scant 2⅓ cups semi-skimmed or skimmed milk. Unlimited tea (including herbal or fruit tea) and mineral water. Glass of pomegranate, blueberry, cranberry or apple juice
Supplements: see page 195

DAILY EXERCISE ROUTINE

Keep up your walking, cycling or swimming routine (see pages 195–196). Do the stretch exercises from the first six days of the program followed by these calf stretches.

CALF STRETCHES

1 Stand comfortably with your feet slightly apart. With your right foot, step forward so that your left heel comes off the ground.
2 Bend your right knee a little and place both hands on your right thigh. Slowly, press your left heel back toward the ground so you feel your left calf stretching. Hold the stretch for a count of five. Repeat the stretch on your right leg.

CONSULTING AN ACUPUNCTURIST

Having followed the full-strength program for one week, you should have noticed an improvement in your arthritis symptoms. It's now time to consult a complementary therapist for individual advice. I suggest you have a course of traditional Chinese acupuncture to complement the acupressure techniques you have been using. Acupuncture can regulate the flow of qi energy in your body to help reduce joint pain and inflammation, and it can improve your range of movement.

During a consultation, the practitioner will ask you about your medical history and examine you physically, which may include an assessment of your tongue and pulse (see page 66). Sterile, disposable, slender needles are inserted into the skin at selected acupoints (this is usually painless, but you may notice a slight pricking, tingling or buzzing sensation). An acupuncturist will use between six and 12 needles, usually on points on the hands and feet. He or she may stimulate the needles with a small, low frequency electrical current or with a burning herb called moxa (this technique is called moxibustion). Some needles are left in position for a few seconds; others may be left for 30 minutes or more. A course of 12 treatments over six weeks can significantly improve your arthritis symptoms. To find an accredited acupuncturist, go to page 234.

DAY EIGHT

DAILY MENU

Breakfast: toast with a scraping of olive-oil spread. Berry and Apple Jelly (see page 222)
Morning snack: Red Delicious apple or a handful of black grapes
Lunch: ½ sliced red pepper. Bowl of mixed bean salad (tinned or homemade). Rye bread. Bowl of mixed red salad leaves with Pecan Nut Oil and Red Wine Vinegar Dressing (see page 225). "High ORAC" fruit (see pages 74–75)
Afternoon snack: handful of walnuts
Dinner: grilled fish fillet with Chilli Chips (see page 208). Sweetcorn. Peas. 40–50g (about 1½oz) bar dark chocolate and/or a handful of cherries
Drinks: 570ml/20fl oz/ scant 2⅓ cups semi-skimmed or skimmed milk. Unlimited tea (including herbal or fruit tea) and mineral water. Glass of pomegranate, blueberry, cranberry or apple juice
Supplements: see page 195

Over the next few days I suggest several different complementary therapies that are beneficial for arthritis. Once you've found a therapy that suits you, find ways to incorporate it into your life.

DAILY EXERCISE ROUTINE

Go walking, cycling or swimming (see pages 195–196). Do your usual sequence of stretches (see days one to seven) followed by today's stretch.

HORIZONTAL FORWARD BENDS

1 Sit on the floor on a comfortable surface such as an exercise mat. Keep your legs together and in front of you.
2 Reach forward and try to touch your toes (or as far down your legs as you can manage). Hold the stretch for a count of 10.

MAGNETIC PATCHES

Today, I'd like you to buy some adhesive magnetic patches and stick two or three on tender points around your most painful joints to improve circulation and promote healing. (Magnetic patches are increasingly used to boost healing of bone fractures.) You may also like to try placing a patch over the Governing Vessel 14 acupoint (see day two). Keep the patches in place for five days, remove them for two days, then reapply.

CHILLI CHIPS

To make the chilli chips for today's dinner, cut four to six Russet potatoes into big chunky chips – leave the skins on. Coat them in chilli oil (simply mix 30ml/ 2fl oz olive oil with two teaspoons of chilli powder). Bake the chips in the oven (200°C/400°F/Gas 6) for 25 minutes until golden. This makes enough chips to serve four.

DAY NINE

DAILY MENU

Breakfast: Apple and Carrot Breakfast Muffins (see page 221)
Morning snack: Red Delicious apple or a handful of black grapes
Lunch: Borscht Soup (see page 224). Wholegrain roll (optional). "High-ORAC" fruit (see pages 74–75)

Afternoon snack: handful of pecans
Dinner: Beef, Black Bean and Chilli Stir-fry (see page 227). Mexican Hot Chilli Sauce, optional (see page 227). Noodles. Low-fat vanilla ice cream with Blueberry and Cranberry Jelly (see page 233)

Drinks: 570ml/20fl oz/ scant 2⅓ cups semi-skimmed or skimmed milk. Unlimited tea (including herbal or fruit tea) and mineral water. Glass of pomegranate, blueberry, cranberry or apple juice
Supplements: see page 195

DAILY EXERCISE ROUTINE

Go for a walk, cycle or swim today as outlined on pages 195–196. Add today's hamstring stretches to the sequence you've learned so far.

HAMSTRING STRETCHES

1 Sit on the floor on a comfortable surface, such as an exercise mat, with your legs straight and spread apart.
2 Bend your right knee out to the side and bring your right foot up against your left knee. Try to keep your right knee in contact with the ground. Keeping your left leg straight, slowly bend forward and try to touch your left ankle or foot. Hold the stretch for a count of 10. Repeat with the other leg.

AROMATHERAPY

Today's complementary technique uses a blend of essential oils that, when massaged into painful joints, can significantly decrease arthritis pain. As described on page 40, add the following oils to 100ml carrier oil: eight drops each of eucalyptus and lavender oils; four drops each of marjoram, peppermint and rosemary oils. Gently massage this oil blend into painful joints daily from now on.

USING A KEYBOARD

When using a keyboard, your shoulders should be relaxed, your upper arms
vertical, your forearms horizontal and your wrists in a neutral, balanced position
– not cocked upward. Ergonomically designed keyboards with specially shaped key
pads and integral wrist rests are available – it's worth investing in one. Also, use a
document holder to minimize neck movement.

DAY TEN

DAILY MENU

Breakfast: Omelette with
Caramelized Sweet
Potato and Red Onions
(see page 222)
Morning snack: Red
Delicious apple or a
handful of black grapes
Lunch: Smoked, Peppered
Mackerel and Beetroot
Salad (see page 226).
Wholegrain roll (optional).

"High-ORAC" fruit
(see pages 74–75).
Afternoon snack: handful
of walnuts
Dinner: Aubergine and
Potato Curry (see page
228). Mexican Hot Chilli
Sauce, optional (see page
227). Turmeric and Almond
Rice (see page 229). Four
large black or red plums

Drinks: 570ml/20fl oz/
scant 2⅓ cups semi-
skimmed or skimmed
milk. Unlimited tea
(including herbal or fruit
tea) and mineral water.
Glass of pomegranate,
blueberry, cranberry or
apple juice
Supplements: see page 195

DAILY EXERCISE ROUTINE

Do the nine stretches you've learned so far, followed by today's stretch.
Walk, cycle or swim as described on pages 195–196.

LOWER BACK STRENGTHENERS

1 Lie on a comfortable but firm surface, such as an exercise mat. Bend
your knees and place your feet flat on the floor and put your hands
behind your head.
2 Now contract the muscles of your lower abdomen and buttocks, so your
pelvis tilts upward and the small of your back flattens against the floor.
3 Hold for a count of five, then relax and repeat five to 10 times.

HERBALISM

Today, I'd like you to start using a herbal medicine to ease your arthritis symptoms. The herb I've selected as most appropriate for the full-strength program is extract of rosehips, which can significantly reduce the pain and stiffness associated with all types of arthritis. Make sure that it's likely to suit you by reading about it on page 42. Start taking a supplement that supplies the equivalent of at least 2,000mg (2g) whole rosehip. Take it once or twice a day, depending on the severity of your joint pain and stiffness.

PROLONGED SQUATTING

Squatting for long periods can increase the risk of developing knee osteoarthritis, and may exacerbate symptoms if you already have it. Avoid squatting during activities such as gardening. (If you kneel instead, always use a padded kneeler or strap-on knee pads.)

DAY ELEVEN

DAILY MENU

Breakfast: Cinnamon Toast (see page 221)
Morning snack: Red Delicious apple or a handful of black grapes
Lunch: sliced avocado, beef tomato and mozzarella cheese arranged on a bed of mixed red salad leaves drizzled with Pecan Nut Oil and Red Wine Vinegar Dressing (see page 225).

Wholegrain roll. "High-ORAC" fruit (see pages 74–75)
Afternoon snack: handful of pecans
Dinner: Baked Whole Fish with Lemon and Herbs (see page 186, moderate program). Baked Russet potato. Bowl of mixed red salad leaves drizzled with Pecan Nut Oil and Red Wine Vinegar Dressing

(see page 225). Chilled Strawberry Soup (see page 232)
Drinks: 570ml/20fl oz/ scant 2⅓ cups semi-skimmed or skimmed milk. Unlimited tea (including herbal or fruit tea) and mineral water. Glass of pomegranate, blueberry, cranberry or apple juice
Supplements: see page 195

This evening, put some prunes in green tea and soak them overnight for tomorrow's breakfast.

DAILY EXERCISE ROUTINE

Continue with your walking, cycling or swimming routine as described on pages 195–196. Do the stretches from days one to ten, then add these leg lifts.

LEG LIFTS 1

1 Lie on your back on a comfortable but firm surface, with your knees bent and your feet flat against the floor. Bring your right knee to your chest.
2 Return your leg to its starting position, then let it lie on the floor, shaking it gently to relax the muscles. Repeat step one, this time raising your left leg.

CHAKRA MEDITATION

This chakra meditation draws healing energy up through your body's seven energy centres (see page 68), which run in a vertical line along the centre of the body. Each chakra is associated with a particular colour. Today, I'd like you to focus on opening each chakra in turn by spending two minutes visualizing the colour associated with it. Start with your

---

CORRECT LIFTING

Never bend and lift at the same time. Instead follow these guidelines for safe lifting techniques.
- Stand close to the load. Position your feet on either side of it.
- Squat down by bending at the knees and hips.
- Grasp the object you're lifting with both hands (not fingers) and keep your elbows tucked in.
- Lean forward slightly and, in one smooth action, straighten your hips and knees while lifting the object (keep it close). To lower an object, do these steps in reverse. Always keep your back straight and don't twist.

base chakra and the colour red. Work up to your crown chakra and the colour white. Imagine that your crown chakra is expanding and giving out a white light that envelops your body in a sphere of healing energy. Visualize this energy becoming concentrated within your most painful joints.

DAY TWELVE

DAILY MENU

Breakfast: prunes soaked in green tea (from day eleven)

Morning snack: Red Delicious apple or a handful of black grapes

Lunch: Kidney bean, Beetroot and Feta Salad (see page 224). Wholegrain roll optional). "High-ORAC" fruit

(see pages 74–75)

Afternoon snack: handful of walnuts

Dinner: Hungarian Goulash (see page 231). Mexican Hot Chilli Sauce, optional (see page 227). Red or brown rice. 40–50g (about 1½oz) bar dark chocolate and/or a handful of raspberries

Drinks: 570ml/20fl oz/ scant 2⅓ cups semi-skimmed or skimmed milk. Unlimited tea (including herbal or fruit tea) and mineral water. Glass of pomegranate, blueberry, cranberry or apple juice

Supplements: see page 195

Cook extra rice for your dinner today – you can eat it in a salad for tomorrow's lunch.

DAILY EXERCISE ROUTINE

Go walking, cycling or swimming (see pages 195–196). Do the stretch exercises from days one to eleven, followed by these leg lifts, which complement the ones from day eleven.

LEG LIFTS 2

1 After you've done yesterday's leg lifts, straighten your right leg and lift it as high as you can off the ground.

2 Lower your right leg slowly and relax. Repeat with your left leg. Practise this five to 10 times on each side.

COPPER THERAPY

Today I'd like you to start using a pair of Copper Heelers (shoe inserts; see page 50). These are available from pharmacies or from www.theoriginalcopperheeler.com. Alternatively, if you haven't already used a copper bracelet (see page 169), start using one now. If you're already using a copper bracelet, put one on the other arm, too.

HOT CHILLI PEPPERS

The heat of chilli peppers is rated using the Scoville scale – consult it whenever you're choosing a chilli for a recipe. The hotter the pepper, the more it will help your arthritis.

- Pure capsaicin: 15,000,000–16,000,000
- Habanero: 350,000–577,000
- Scotch Bonnet: 100,000–350,000
- Jamaican hot pepper: 100,000–200,000
- Thai pepper: 50,000–100,000
- Cayenne pepper, Tabasco pepper: 30,000–50,000
- Serrano pepper: 10,000–23,000

- Tabasco sauce: 7,000–8,000
- Wax pepper: 5,000–10,000
- Jalapeño pepper: 2,500–8,000
- Rocotillo pepper: 1,500–2,500
- Poblano pepper: 1,000–1,500
- Anaheim pepper: 500–1,000
- Pimento and pepperoncini: 100–500
- Bell pepper: 0

DAY THIRTEEN

DAILY EXERCISE ROUTINE

Keep up your walking, cycling or swimming regime, as outlined on pages 195–196. Remember to warm up and cool down first. Do the stretch exercises from the previous days, followed by these pelvic circles.

PELVIC CIRCLES

1 Lie on your back on a comfortable but firm surface, such as an exercise mat. Hug your knees in to your chest with a hand on each knee.

DAILY MENU

Breakfast: Apple, Kiwi and Blueberry Smoothie (see page 223)
Morning snack: Red Delicious apple or a handful of black grapes
Lunch: Spiced Lentil Salad (see page 226). Tinned tuna with chopped tomato, parsley and low-fat mayonnaise. Bowl of red salad leaves drizzled with Pecan Nut Oil and Red Wine Vinegar Dressing (see page 225). Focaccia. "High-ORAC" fruit (see pages 74–75)
Afternoon snack: handful of pecans
Dinner: pasta with red pesto. Chopped tomato and red onion. Bowl of mixed red salad leaves drizzled with Macadamia Nut and Lemon Juice Dressing (see page 186) and sprinkled with Parmesan shavings and mixed seeds. Peach Melba with Pecans (see page 232)
Drinks: 570ml/20fl oz/ scant 2⅓ cups semi-skimmed or skimmed milk. Unlimited tea (including herbal or fruit tea) and mineral water. Glass of pomegranate, blueberry, cranberry or apple juice
Supplements: see page 195

2 Keep your feet and knees together and draw circles in the air with your knees (near to your chest). Do 10 circles in one direction, then 10 in the opposite direction.

MUD BATH

Today, I'd like you to use some Dead Sea mineral mud (available from pharmacies) in the bath. Draw a deep bath that is hot enough to make the bathroom steamy. Massage the thick, black mud into your most painful joints and add any excess mud to the bath water. Get into the bath and soak for at least 20 minutes in the mineral-rich water. Rinse off in the shower. If you wish, you can reapply the black mineral mud to your most

KEEP MOVING
Muscles and joints need oxygen to retain their flexibility. When they stay in the same position for a length of time they become fatigued and lacking in oxygen, and this triggers pain. Take regular movement breaks at least every 10 to 15 minutes to help maintain muscle and joint mobility.

painful joints, then wrap a bandage around each joint and leave on as a healing poultice for up to 24 hours.

DAY FOURTEEN

DAILY MENU

Breakfast: high-fibre cereal and semi-skimmed milk sprinkled with fresh blueberries
Morning snack: Red Delicious apple or a handful of black grapes
Lunch: ½ avocado with prawns and chopped coriander leaves. Red salad leaves with Pecan Nut Oil and Red Wine Vinegar Dressing (see

page 225). Focaccia or garlic and herb bread. "High ORAC" fruit (see pages 74–75)
Afternoon snack: handful of walnuts
Dinner: Salmon with Pink Peppercorns and Red Lentils (see page 230). Mashed Russet potatoes. Bowl of mixed red leaves with Pecan Nut Oil and Red Wine Vinegar

Dressing (see page 225). Stewed apples and raspberries
Drinks: 570ml/20fl oz/ scant 2⅓ cups semi-skimmed or skimmed milk. Unlimited tea (including herbal or fruit tea) and mineral water. Glass of pomegranate, blueberry, cranberry or apple juice
Supplements: see page 195

DAILY EXERCISE ROUTINE

Keep up your walking, cycling or swimming routine, as described on pages 195–196. As always, remember to warm up and cool down. Do the stretch exercises from days one to thirteen, then add the following hip circles.

HIP CIRCLES

1 Lie on your back in the same starting position as step one of yesterday's pelvic circles.
2 Keeping your feet together, make circles with your knees. Each knee should go in the opposite direction to the other and as wide as possible to the side before coming back in to complete each circle. Do 10 circles like this, then reverse direction and do another 10 with each knee circling in the opposite direction.

CONSULTING A REIKI MASTER

Having followed the full-strength plan for two weeks, it's now time to consult a holistic practitioner, and I suggest you experience spiritual healing with a Reiki master. Reiki healing channels universal energy through the chakra centres on which you meditated on day eleven (see pages 212–213). A treatment session lasts around an hour, during which you lie clothed on a table. The practitioner holds his or her hands on or over your body in 12 basic positions for five minutes each: four of these are on your head, four on the front of your body and four on the back. You may feel heat emanating from the healer's hands. You may feel relaxed or sometimes invigorated after a Reiki session. To find a practitioner, see the resources on page 235.

CONTINUING THE FULL-STRENGTH PROGRAM

Well done – you have followed the full-strength program for 14 days. Now I'd like you to repeat the program so that it lasts for a full 28 days. Eating a diet that is so high in antioxidants (20,000 ORAC units a day or more) should significantly ease your arthritis symptoms. If this is the case, apply the principles of the program every day from now on.

If the full-strength program doesn't provide symptom relief, and you've already tried the previous programs, it's likely that some other component of your diet apart from an imbalance between omega-6s and omega-3s, or exposure to nightshade plants is affecting your joint symptoms. You may wish to try excluding meat from your diet (see page 79), or acid-forming foods (see pages 79–81), or to follow a full elimination-and-challenge diet. An elimination-and-challenge diet involves excluding foods to which you suspect you may have an intolerance. In surveys, the foods most likely to provoke arthritis symptoms are: bacon, beef, caffeine, corn, dairy products, grapefruit, lamb, lemons, malt, oranges, pork, rye, sugar, tomatoes, wheat and yeast.

You may wish to exclude all these from your diet to see if your symptoms improve. You can then reintroduce eliminated foods one by one, usually at three-day intervals, to see if they provoke symptoms. Here's how a suspect food is typically reintroduced:

• DAY 1

Breakfast: eat a small quantity of test food (for example, 30g/1oz cheese). Monitor for adverse reactions over four hours. If OK:
Lunch: eat twice the amount eaten that morning (for example, 60g/2oz cheese). Monitor for adverse reactions over 4 hours. If OK:
Dinner: eat twice the amount eaten at lunch (for example, 120g/4oz cheese).

• DAY 2

Eat a basic elimination diet (consisting of foods you know don't upset your symptoms). Avoid the test food. Monitor for delayed reactions to the test food.

• DAY 3

Assess whether or not your symptoms are worse as a result of eating the test food. If an adverse reaction occurs, continue to avoid the test food and wait 48 hours after all symptoms have gone before testing another food. If the results are unclear, repeat the steps from day one, but using larger doses of the suspect food. If the suspect food does not worsen your symptoms, you can add it to the list of foods that you can eat. You can start testing a new food on day four using the same method.

Although you can try this on your own at home, it's best to follow a full elimination-and-challenge diet under the supervision of a naturopath or nutritionist who is experienced in diagnosing food intolerances. Another approach is to have a blood test that assesses the way your white blood cells react to a variety of different food extracts, or to measure your levels of IgG anti-food antibodies. These tests (see page 77) are at least 70 percent effective in pinpointing culprit foods.

YOUR LONG-TERM DIET

If you opt to stay on the full-strength program, continue to eat lots of fresh fruit and vegetables, selected nuts and oily fish to maximize your intake of anti-inflammatory antioxidants. Go back and read pages 72–75 – about the high-ORAC diet – to refresh your memory of the highest scoring fruit and vegetables.

RECIPES

Continue to explore recipes containing high antioxidant foods, especially fish-based and vegetarian recipes. You will find some recipe suggestions at www.naturalhealthguru.co.uk and you can post your own favourites there, too, for other followers of the full-strength program to try.

YOUR LONG-TERM SUPPLEMENT REGIME

Continue taking the recommended supplements (see page 195) long term. Research supports their use at this high level for significant beneficial effects on joint health. If, up until now, you have taken only the supplements in the recommended list, you may also wish to add in one or more from the optional list for extra benefit. Alternatively, if your arthritis symptoms are well controlled, you may wish to reduce the dose of your supplements back down to the levels suggested in the moderate program and see if this lower dose remains beneficial.

YOUR EXERCISE ROUTINE

After performing the full-strength exercises for four weeks, you should notice an improvement in muscle strength and joint flexibility. Continue doing these stretch and range-of-motion exercises, ideally twice a day. Also try to fit in some walking, cycling or swimming, building up to 30 to 40 minutes most days of the week. Consider starting other activities such as dancing, gardening, bowling or golf, too.

YOUR THERAPY PROGRAM

The full-strength program has shown you how to use acupressure to ease your joint symptoms, and has introduced you to several other

DIAGNOSTIC TECHNIQUES FOR FOOD INTOLERANCE
There is little evidence to support the use of VEGA electrodermal testing, applied kinesiology (muscle strength) testing or hair mineral analysis and I don't personally recommend these. Having said that, a few people have undoubtedly found them helpful.

complementary techniques, including aromatherapy, magnetic patches, copper, Dead Sea mineral mud, herbal medicine and meditation. Continue using the therapies that you have found beneficial, and continue to consult the acupuncturist and Reiki healer I suggested you see on days seven and fourteen if you found their treatments helpful. You may also want to explore some of the other therapies I mentioned in Part Two, such as chiropractic or osteopathy.

MONITORING YOUR JOINT SYMPTOMS

From now on, I suggest you continue to monitor and score your joint symptoms at least once a month, to make sure you continue to show some benefits. If your joint scores stop showing an improvement, or if they start to worsen again, check you are taking the level of supplements I recommend as desirable for the full-strength program and consider taking one or more of those I give as options for additional health benefits (see page 195). If your joint symptoms remain troublesome, I suggest you visit a naturopath or nutritionist to receive individually tailored advice about your diet.

BREAKFAST RECIPES

APPLE AND CARROT BREAKFAST MUFFINS

SERVES 4

100g/3½oz mixed, dried fruit, for example, blueberries, cranberries, raisins, chopped prunes and chopped dates

100g/3½oz/1 cup pecan nuts, chopped

85g/3oz/½ cup plus 1 tbsp plain wholemeal flour

80g/2¾oz/¾ cup rolled oats

30g/1oz/⅓ cup dried skimmed milk powder

1½ tsp baking powder

1 tsp ground cinnamon

1 tsp ground ginger

2 omega-3-enriched eggs, lightly beaten

125ml/4fl oz/½ cup olive oil

3 tbsp clear honey

3 tbsp maple syrup

1 tsp vanilla extract

1 large Red Delicious apple, grated

100g/3½oz carrots, peeled and grated

1 Preheat the oven to 180°C/350°F/Gas 4.

2 Mix together the dried fruit, pecan nuts, flour, oats, milk powder, baking powder, cinnamon and ginger in a bowl.

3 In a separate bowl, beat together the eggs, oil, honey, maple syrup and vanilla essence. Add the apple and carrot, and then the flour mixture from the first bowl.

4 Mix briefly with a large spoon. Spoon into 8 large muffin cases, and bake for 20 minutes. Serve warm or cool.

CINNAMON TOAST

SERVES 4

4 slices wholemeal bread

1 tsp freshly ground cinnamon

1 tsp golden caster sugar

40g/1½oz butter

1 Toast the bread on one side. Mix together the cinnamon, sugar and butter.

2 Butter the untoasted side then place under a low grill until evenly brown. Cut into fingers and serve hot.

BERRY AND APPLE JELLY

MAKES 3 JARS

900g/2lb/7 cups fresh berries, for
   example, raspberries, strawberries,
   blueberries or blackberries, rinsed
3 Red Delicious apples, chopped
   (including skin, core and pips)
Juice and pips of 2 lemons
700g/1lb 9oz/scant 3¼ cups
   granulated sugar

1 Preheat the oven to 180°C/350°F/Gas
   4. Sterilize 3 x 225g/8oz jam jars and
   lids by heating them in the oven for
   15 minutes.

2 Put all the fruit, juice and pips in a
   stainless steel jam pan. Add enough
   water to cover the fruit and cook on
   top of the stove until the mixture is
   soft. Pour into a muslin bag and hang
   over a non-metallic bowl overnight,
   to catch the juice (or pass through
   a conical sieve).

3 Pour the juice into a measuring jug
   and record the volume. For every
   600ml/21fl oz/2½ cups you need to
   add 450g/1lb/2 cups sugar.

4 Put the juices and sugar in a clean
   jam pan and heat gently to dissolve
   the sugar. Boil rapidly until the jelly
   reaches setting point (105°C/220°F).
   Remove from the heat and skim off
   any froth, then pour into the jars and
   seal with lids. Label and store in a
   cool, dry, place.

OMELETTE WITH CARAMELIZED SWEET POTATO AND RED ONIONS

SERVES 4

2 tbsp olive oil
1 red onion, thinly sliced
1 sweet potato, peeled and grated
1 garlic clove, chopped
1 sprig oregano leaves, chopped
1 tbsp maple syrup or clear honey
8 omega-3-enriched eggs
1 handful grated cheese, for example,
   Cheddar, mozzarella, Gruyère
Freshly ground black pepper

1 Heat half of the olive oil in a
   saucepan and sauté the onion, sweet
   potato, garlic and oregano. Add the
   maple syrup or honey and cook for
   a further 2 minutes. Keep stirrring.

2 Beat the eggs lightly and season with
   black pepper. Heat the remaining
   olive oil in an omelette pan over high
   heat. Tip in the eggs, cook until
   there's only a little runny egg left,
   then remove from the heat.

3 Sprinkle the sweet potato and onion
   over one half of the omelette. Add the
   cheese. Season with black pepper.

4 Return to the heat for 30 seconds.
   Flip the uncovered side of the
   omelette over, slide onto a plate
   and serve.

APPLE, KIWI AND BLUEBERRY SMOOTHIE
SERVES 4

4 red eating apples, cored
4 kiwi fruit, peeled
300g/10½oz blueberries
100ml/3½fl oz/scant ½ cup
  unsweetened apple juice

1 Whiz the fruit in a blender then stir in
   the apple juice slowly (using more or
   less juice to create the consistency
   you like).

APPLE AND RASPBERRY SMOOTHIE
SERVES 4

4 red eating apples, cored
300g/10½oz raspberries
100ml/3½fl oz/scant ½ cup
  unsweetened apple juice

1 Whiz the fruit in a blender then stir in
   the apple juice slowly (using more or
   less juice to create the consistency
   you like).

LUNCH RECIPES

KIDNEY BEAN, BEETROOT AND FETA SALAD

SERVES 4

400g/14oz/2 cups cooked kidney beans
1 beetroot, cooked, peeled and grated
1 carrot, peeled and grated
1 red onion, chopped
4 tomatoes, chopped
100g/3½oz/⅔ cup crumbled feta
  cheese
1 red lettuce, for example, lollo rosso
  or red oak leaf, chopped

For the dressing:
4 tbsp walnut oil
1 garlic clove, crushed
1 tbsp red wine vinegar
1 handful chopped herbs, for example,
  basil and parsley
Freshly ground black pepper

1 Put the dressing ingredients in a small
   jar with a screwtop lid and shake.
2 Mix the salad ingredients together
   and pour the dressing over the top.
   Toss and serve immediately.

BORSCHT SOUP

SERVES 4

1 tbsp olive oil
1 red onion, chopped
1 garlic clove, crushed
1 large celery stick, chopped
1 small fennel bulb, chopped
5 beetroot, peeled and grated
600ml/21fl oz/2½ cups vegetable stock
  or water
2 tomatoes, skinned
1 handful baby spinach leaves
Zest and juice of 1 unwaxed lemon
1 tbsp chopped basil
4 tbsp crème fraîche or low-fat
  bio yogurt
Freshly ground black pepper

1 Heat the olive oil in a pan and sauté
   the onion, garlic, celery and fennel for
   10 minutes. Add the beetroot and
   cover with the stock. Simmer for 5
   minutes, then add the tomatoes and
   cook for another 5 minutes. Add the
   spinach leaves, lemon zest and juice,
   and cook for a further 2 minutes.
2 Purée in a blender until smooth.
   Season with plenty of black pepper.
   Serve hot or cold in four bowls with a
   sprinkling of basil and a tablespoon of
   crème fraîche in each.

SALMON AND MIXED BEAN LUNCH BOWL

SERVES 4

4 Russet potatoes
1 red lettuce, for example, lollo rosso
    or red oak leaf, shredded
600g/1lb 5oz/3 cups mixed cooked
    beans, for example, red kidney beans,
    chickpeas or black beans
400g/14oz cold, cooked salmon
    (poached, grilled or roasted), flaked
1 red onion, chopped
1 slice red cabbage, shredded
½ cucumber, chopped
1 handful cherry tomatoes
1 handful chopped parsley

For the dressing:
4 tbsp walnut oil
1 garlic clove, crushed
1 tbsp red wine vinegar
1 tbsp chopped herbs, for example,
    parsley or coriander
Freshly ground black pepper

1 Boil the potatoes in their skins until
    cooked. Allow to cool until warm and
    chop into chunks.
2 Put the dressing ingredients in a
    screwtop jar and shake. Mix together
    all the salad ingredients and pour the
    dressing over the top. Toss and serve
    immediately.

PECAN NUT OIL AND RED WINE VINEGAR DRESSING

SERVES 4

6 tbsp pecan nut oil
2 tbsp red wine vinegar (or raspberry
    vinegar)
Freshly ground black pepper

1 Put the ingredients in a screwtop jar
    and shake. Store the dressing in a
    cool, dry place – it will keep for
    several days.

SPICED LENTIL SALAD

SERVES 4

225g/8oz/scant 1 cup red lentils
1 red onion, finely chopped
2 garlic cloves, crushed
2½cm/1in piece root ginger, peeled and
  finely chopped
1 tsp cumin seeds, crushed
1 tbsp coriander seeds, crushed
4 tbsp olive oil
1 large carrot, grated
Zest and juice of 1 unwaxed lemon
1 handful chopped coriander leaves
4 little gem lettuce hearts
Freshly ground black pepper

1 Simmer the lentils in 600ml/21fl oz/
   scant 2½ cups water for 30 minutes,
   until tender. Drain.

2 Sauté the onion, garlic, ginger, cumin
   and coriander seeds in olive oil. Add
   the spiced onion mixture, carrot,
   and lemon zest and juice to the
   lentils. Stir.

3 Season with black pepper and
   sprinkle with coriander leaves.
   Serve warm or chilled on top of
   the lettuce leaves.

SMOKED, PEPPERED MACKEREL AND BEETROOT SALAD

SERVES 4

100g/3½oz/¾ cup green beans, topped
  and tailed
1 red lettuce, for example, lollo rosso or
  red oak leaf, shredded
1 small beetroot, peeled and grated
Zest and juice of 1 unwaxed lemon
2 tbsp extra virgin olive oil
4 fillets smoked mackerel with black
  peppercorns

For the dressing:
4 tbsp low-fat bio yogurt
2 tsp clear honey
1 tbsp wholegrain mustard
1 handful chopped dill

1 Blanch the green beans in boiling
   water for 1 minute. Drain, refresh
   under cold running water and dry.

2 Put the dressing ingredients in a
   screwtop jar and shake.

3 Toss the lettuce, beetroot and beans
   in the lemon zest and juice and olive
   oil. Divide between 4 plates and put a
   mackerel fillet on top of each. Pour
   the dressing over the top.

DINNER RECIPES

MEXICAN HOT CHILLI SAUCE
SERVES 4

2 tbsp olive oil

1 red onion, finely chopped

1 tsp ground cumin

2 garlic cloves, crushed

2 carrots, grated

1 handful chopped oregano

4 hot red chillies (habaneros), deseeded and finely chopped

Zest and juice of 2 unwaxed limes

2 tbsp red wine vinegar

1 Heat the oil in a pan and sauté the onion, cumin and garlic until the onions are soft. Add the carrots, 250ml/9fl oz/1 cup water and oregano and bring to the boil. Simmer gently until the carrots are soft.

2 Add the chillies, lime zest and juice and vinegar. Purée in a blender until smooth.

BEEF, BLACK BEAN AND CHILLI STIR-FRY
SERVES 4

450g/1lb lean fillet beef, cut into thin strips

2 red onions, thinly sliced

2 garlic cloves, chopped

1 red chilli, finely chopped

2 tbsp olive oil

250g/9oz baby spinach leaves, washed

1 head of broccoli, cut into florets

1 green pepper, deseeded and chopped

½ cucumber, cut into thin strips

200g/7oz black bean sauce

1 Stir-fry the beef, onions, garlic and chilli in olive oil until browned. Add the spinach, broccoli, green pepper and cucumber. Cook for 3 minutes.

2 Stir in the black bean sauce and heat through for 1 minute before serving immediately.

RED LENTIL DHAL

SERVES 4

225g/8oz/scant 1 cup red lentils, washed
4 tbsp olive oil
1 red onion, chopped
1 garlic clove, crushed
1 tbsp coriander seed, ground
1 tsp ground cumin
1 tsp turmeric
1 tsp fenugreek seeds, ground
1 tsp chilli powder
2½cm/1in piece ginger, peeled and
   grated
4 tbsp red wine vinegar
1 handful chopped coriander leaves

1 Cook the lentils in 600ml/21fl oz/
   scant 2½ cups water according to the
   packet instructions. Drain, retaining
   the cooking liquid.

2 Heat the oil in a pan and sauté the
   onion and garlic until they start to
   colour.

3 Mix together the spices and red wine
   vinegar to make a thick paste. Add
   the spice paste to the onion mixture
   and gently sauté for 5 minutes. Add
   the drained lentils, coriander and
   some of the cooking liquid to obtain
   your preferred thickness.

AUBERGINE AND POTATO CURRY

SERVES 4

2 tsp cumin seeds
2 tsp mustard seeds
4 tbsp olive oil
2 red onions, chopped
300g/11oz aubergine, cubed
55g/2oz/¼ cup red lentils
200ml/7fl oz/scant 1 cup vegetable
   stock
1 tsp turmeric
1 tbsp desiccated coconut
2 green chillies, slit lengthways
2½cm/1in piece root ginger, peeled
   and finely chopped
1 tsp chilli powder
2 tsp ground coriander
1 handful chopped coriander leaves

1 Sauté the cumin and mustard seeds
   in the oil until they start to crackle.
   Add the onions and stir-fry until soft.

2 Add all the remaining ingredients,
   cover and simmer gently until all
   the vegetables are cooked (15–20
   minutes). Stir occasionally and, if the
   curry becomes too dry, add more
   water. Serve sprinkled with the
   coriander leaves.

TURMERIC AND ALMOND RICE

SERVES 4

225g/8oz/heaped 1 cup long-grain rice,
  for example, Basmati
2 tsp turmeric
300ml/10½fl oz/scant 1¼ cups coconut
  milk
1 large handful almond flakes
1 handful chopped parsley or coriander
  leaves

1 Boil the rice in 455ml/16fl oz/1¾ cups
   water, then simmer gently until the
   water is absorbed.

2 Add the turmeric to the coconut milk
   and stir well before pouring over the
   rice.

3 Simmer the rice until the milk is
   absorbed. Put on a serving dish, add
   the almond flakes and fluff up with a
   fork. Serve sprinkled with parsley or
   coriander.

SAFFRON RICE

SERVES 4

1 large pinch saffron stamens
4 tbsp olive oil
1l/35fl oz/4 cups boiling stock
1 large red onion, chopped
2 garlic cloves, crushed
2 pieces cinnamon stick
4 whole cloves
10 cardamom pods, seeds only
375g/13oz/1¾ cups long-grain rice
1 handful chopped parsley or coriander
  leaves

1 Cover the saffron with 3 tablespoons
   of boiling stock and soak for 10
   minutes.

2 Heat the oil in the pan and sauté the
   onions, garlic, cinnamon, cloves and
   cardamom seeds. Add the rice and
   stir for 5 minutes.

3 Add the remaining stock and bring to
   the boil. Add the saffron and its
   soaking water. Cover and simmer for
   25 minutes. Drain and serve with
   parsley or coriander.

MANGO SALSA SALMON STEAKS

SERVES 4

4 salmon fillets
1 tbsp olive oil

For the salsa:
1 mango, flesh finely chopped
1 Red Delicious apple, finely chopped
  with skin on
Zest and juice of 1 unwaxed lime
1 red chilli, deseeded and finely chopped
1 handful chopped coriander leaves

1 Mix the salsa ingredients and
   marinate in the fridge for at least
   1 hour.

2 Brush the salmon fillets with olive oil
   and grill until the flesh is set. Serve
   the salmon with the mango salsa on
   the side.

SALMON WITH PINK PEPPERCORNS AND RED LENTILS

SERVES 4

4 salmon fillets
3 tbsp olive oil
225g/8oz/scant 1 cup red lentils, rinsed
2 red onions, chopped
1 garlic clove, crushed
2 tsp pink peppercorns
1 heaped tbsp crème fraîche
1 handful chopped basil leaves
Freshly ground black pepper

1 Preheat the oven to 160°C/325°F/Gas 3.

2 Put the salmon in an ovenproof dish,
   drizzle with 1 tablespoon of olive oil
   and season well with black pepper.
   Cover with silver foil and roast for
   15 minutes until the flesh has just set.

3 Cook the red lentils in 600ml/21fl
   oz/2½ cups of water according
   to the packet instructions. Heat
   1 tablespoon of olive oil in a pan
   and sauté the red onion and garlic
   until just soft.

4 Stir in the pink peppercorns, crème
   fraîche and basil. Drain the lentils
   and toss in 1 tablespoon of olive oil.
   Divide between 4 plates. Put a
   fillet of salmon and some sauce
   on top of each.

HUNGARIAN GOULASH

SERVES 4

1 tbsp olive oil

3 red onions, chopped

2 garlic cloves, crushed

1 green pepper, deseeded and chopped

1 red pepper, deseeded and chopped

450g/1lb lean stewing steak, cut into
  small chunks

1 tbsp sweet paprika

2 tsp hot paprika

4 tomatoes, chopped

2 tbsp tomato purée

2 bay leaves

150ml/5fl oz/scant ⅔ cup vegetable
  stock or water

150ml/5fl oz/scant ⅔ cup red wine

3 unpeeled Russet potatoes, cubed

Zest and juice of 1 unwaxed lemon

Freshly ground black pepper

1 Preheat the oven to 150°C/300°F/Gas 2.

2 Heat the olive oil in a pan and sauté
   the onions, garlic and peppers until
   the onions are golden. Add the meat
   and cook for 5 minutes, while stirring.
   Add the paprikas, tomatoes, tomato
   purée, bay leaves, stock and wine.

3 Transfer to a casserole dish and cook
   for 2 hours. Add the potatoes, lemon
   zest and juice, and cook for a further
   hour. Season well with black pepper.

EXTRA-SPICY CHILLI BEANS

SERVES 4

250g/9oz dried kidney beans (soaked
  overnight and rinsed)

1 tbsp olive oil

2 red onions, chopped

4 garlic cloves, crushed

4 carrots, grated

2 red peppers, deseeded and chopped

2 celery sticks, finely chopped

2 tsp ground cumin

6 tsp ground coriander

2 red chillies, chopped

8 ripe tomatoes, chopped

2 tbsp tomato purée

150ml/5fl oz/scant ⅔ cup red wine

Zest and juice of 1 unwaxed lemon

55g/2oz/⅓ cup bulgur wheat

1 handful chopped coriander leaves

Freshly ground black pepper

1 Simmer the beans in 1.25l/44fl oz/5
   cups water for 60 minutes. Drain and
   retain the cooking liquid.

2 Heat the oil in a pan and sauté the
   red onions and garlic, then add the
   carrots, peppers, celery, beans and
   spices. Cook for 5 minutes.

3 Add the tomatoes, tomato purée, red
   wine, lemon zest and juice, bulgur
   wheat and about 600ml/21fl oz/2½
   cups of the retained liquid. Simmer
   for 40 minutes.

4 Add the coriander leaves and extra
   liquid. Cover and cook for another
   20 minutes. Season with black pepper
   and serve.

DESSERT RECIPES

FRESH STRAWBERRY COULIS
SERVES 4

500g/1lb 2oz/3⅓ cups strawberries,
   hulled and halved
1 tbsp icing sugar
Low-fat vanilla ice-cream, to serve

1 Put the ingredients in a metal bowl,
   add 2 tbsp water and cover. Place
   over a pan of simmering water for
   90 minutes then strain the juice.
   Serve with the ice-cream.

PEACH MELBA WITH PECANS
SERVES 4

85g/3oz/½ cup golden caster sugar
1 vanilla pod (or 2 tsp vanilla extract)
4 peaches, peeled and halved
225g/8oz/1¾ cups raspberries
55g/2oz/scant ½ cup icing sugar
1 handful pecan nuts, chopped

1 Put the sugar, vanilla pod and
   300ml/10½fl oz/scant 1¼ cups water
   in a pan and simmer, stirring, until the
   sugar dissolves. Poach the peaches in
   the syrup for 5 minutes.
2 Whiz the raspberries and icing sugar
   in a blender. Add a little water (or
   some of the syrup) to make a coulis.
   Serve the cooled peaches with the
   coulis and sprinkle with the pecans.

CHILLED STRAWBERRY SOUP
SERVES 4

500g/1lb 2oz/3⅓ cups strawberries,
   hulled and halved
1 tbsp golden caster sugar
125ml/4fl oz/½ cup light red wine,
   for example, Beaujolais
Zest and juice of 2 unwaxed oranges
Zest and juice of 1 unwaxed lemon
Freshly ground black pepper

1 Put the strawberries in a bowl
   (reserving a few) and sprinkle with
   the sugar and a little black pepper.
   Leave to marinate.
2 Pour the wine into a saucepan, add
   the fruit zest, the lemon juice and
   half the orange juice, then bring to
   the boil. Simmer, uncovered, until the
   volume has reduced by half. Strain
   and leave until cold.
3 Stir the wine into the strawberries
   and add the remaining orange juice.
   Whiz in a blender. Season with black
   pepper. Serve with the reserved
   strawberries.

CHOCOLATE, PRUNE AND PECAN SQUARES

SERVES 8

55g/2oz dark chocolate (at least
  70 percent cocoa solids)
15g/½oz butter
55g/2oz/¼ cup semi-dried prunes,
  chopped and soaked overnight in
  black or green tea
55g/2oz/½ cup pecan nuts, chopped
2 omega-3-enriched eggs
225g/8oz/scant 1 cup Demerara sugar
55g/2oz/scant ½ cup self-raising flour

1 Preheat the oven to 180°C/350°F/
   Gas 4.

2 Melt the chocolate and butter in a
   metal bowl over simmering water.
   Remove from heat and stir in all
   the remaining ingredients.

3 Pour into a non-stick baking tin
   (25.5 x 15cm/10 x 6in) lined with
   baking paper. Bake for 30 minutes.
   Cool and cut into squares.

BLUEBERRY AND CRANBERRY JELLY

SERVES 4

175g/6oz/1 cup blueberries, fresh or
  thawed from frozen
500ml/17fl oz/2 cups cranberry juice
11g/¼oz gelatine powder
4 handfuls fresh mixed berries, for
  example, strawberries and raspberries

1 Put the blueberries and half the
   cranberry juice in a saucepan and
   bring to the boil. Simmer gently for
   2 minutes.

2 Heat the rest of the cranberry juice
   until it bubbles, then sprinkle in the
   gelatine powder, stirring briskly, until
   it dissolves. Pour into the blueberry
   mixture and mix well.

3 Rinse out a jelly mould with cold
   water, then pour in the jelly. Allow
   to cool, stirring occasionally. Leave
   in the fridge to set.

4 To turn out the jelly, dip the mould
   in hot water, invert onto a plate and
   tap the bottom. Serve with the
   mixed berries.

RESOURCES

Visit **www.naturalhealthguru.co.uk** for more information, medical references and to post comments and questions about the programs.

Arthritis
- Arthritis UK
  www.arthritiscare.org.uk
- Arthritic Assocation (UK)
  www.arthriticassociation.org.uk
- Arthritis Research Campaign (UK)
  www.arc.org.uk
- UK Gout Society
  www.ukgoutsociety.org
- National Rheumatoid Arthritis Society (UK)
  www.rheumatoid.org.uk
- Arthritis Australia
  www.arthritisaustralia.com.au
- Australian Rheumatology Association
  www.rheumatology.org.au
- Arthritis New Zealand
  www.arthritis.org.nz

Complementary Medicine Associations
- Australian Traditional Medicine Society
  www.atms.com.au
- British Complementary Medicine Association
  www.bcma.co.uk
- New Zealand Natural Medicine Association
  www.nznma.com
- UK Complementary Medical Association
  www.the-cma.org.uk

- UK Institute for Complementary Medicine
  www.i-c-m.org.uk

Acupuncture and acupressure
- Australian Acupuncture and Oriental Medicine Alliance
  www.aomalliance.org
- British Acupuncture Council
  www.acupuncture.org.uk
- British Medical Acupuncture Society
  www.medical-acupuncture.co.uk

Aromatherapy
- Australia: International Federation of Aromatherapists
  www.ifa.org.au
- International Federation of Professional Aromatherapists
  www.ifparoma.org

Chiropractic and osteopathy
- British Chiropractic Association
  www.chiropractic-uk.co.uk
- McTimoney Chiropractic Association (UK)
  www.mctimoney-chiropractic.org
- General Chiropractic Council (UK)
  www.gcc-uk.org
- Chiropractors' Association of Australia
  www.chiropractors.asn.au
- New Zealand Chiropractors' Association
  www.chiropractic.org.nz
- World Federation of Chiropractic
  www.wfc.org
- Australian Osteopathic Association
  www.osteopathic.com.au

- British Osteopathic Association
  www.osteopathy.org
- General Osteopathic Council, UK
  www.osteopathy.org.uk
- Osteopathic Council of New Zealand
  www.osteopathiccouncilorg.nz

Food intolerance
- Allergy UK
  www.allergyuk.org
- World Allergy Organization
  www.worldallergy.org
- Allergy New Zealand
  www.allergy.org.nz
- Allergy Society of Australia
  www.allergy.org.au

Herbal medicine
- International Register of Consultant
  Herbalists and Homeopaths
  www.irch.org
- UK National Institute of Medical
  Herbalists
  www.nimh.org.uk
- National Herbalists Association of
  Australia
  www.nhaa.org.au

Homeopathy
- Australian Homoeopathic Association
  www.homeopathyoz.org
- Faculty of Homeopathy (UK)
  www.trusthomeopathy.org
- International Register of Consultant
  Herbalists and Homeopaths
  www.irch.org

Naturopathy
- Australian Naturopathic Practitioners
  Association
  www.anpa.asn.au
- British Naturopathic Association
  www.naturopaths.org.uk

Qigong
- Tai Chi Australia
  www.taichiaustralia.com.au
- Tai Chi Union for Great Britain
  www.taichiunion.com

Reflexology
- Association of Reflexologists (UK)
  www.aor.org.uk
- British Reflexology Association
  www.britreflex.co.uk
- Reflexology Association of Australia
  www.reflexology.org.au

Reiki
- UK Reiki Federation
  www.reikifed.co.uk
- Australian Reiki Connection
  www.australianreikiconnection.com.au
- Reiki New Zealand
  www.reiki.org.nz

Yoga
- British Wheel of Yoga
  www.bwy.org.uk
- Yoga Centers Australia
  www.yoga-centers-directory.net

INDEX

chicken
 chicken, lime and grape
  salad 143
 mildly spiced grilled
  chicken 146
chilli peppers 83, 192–4, 214
 beef, black bean and chilli
  stir-fry 227
 chilli chips 208
 extra-spicy chilli beans 231
 mexican hot chilli sauce
  227
 sweet chilli jelly 145
chiropractic, development of
 56–8
chiropractor, consulting
 57–8, 175–6
chocolate
 chocolate cinnamon pecan
  brownies 150
 chocolate lava pudding 191
 chocolate, prune and
  pecan squares 233
 cinnamon chocolate nut
  terrine 190
chondroitin sulphate 92
cinnamon
 chocolate cinnamon pecan
  brownies 150
 cinnamon chocolate nut
  terrine 140
 cinnamon toast 221
coconut
 mild prawn and coconut
  curry 145
cod in soy sauce 147
cod liver oil 91
copper therapy 48–51, 169,
 214
corticosteroids 30
cranberries
 blueberry and cranberry
  jelly 233
 mulled cranberry apples
  151
craniosacral therapy 57
curry
 mild prawn and coconut
  curry 155

disease-modifying
 anti-rheumatic drugs 31–2

elimination and challenge
 diet 71, 76, 217–18
essential oils 39–41
evening primrose oil
 90–91
exercise 8, 97–103
 cooling down 103
 discomfort, dealing with
  99
 full-strength program
  195–6, 219
 gentle program 116–17,
  139
 moderate program
  155, 178–9
 types of 100–102
 warming up 102–3

fennel
 pasta with smoked salmon
  and fennel 189
figs
 figs in red wine 149
 fresh figs with blueberries
  180
finger exercises 125, 169
finger joints, arthritis
 affecting 25
fish
 baked whole fish with
  lemon and herbs 186
 mildly tikka fish 146
 oily 70–71, 85, 138
floatation therapy 47
fluid, drinking 71
folate 88
food intolerance, diagnostic
 techniques 217–19
food sensitivities 158
forward stretches 197–8
fruit
 dark blue-red pigmented
  83
 eating 70
 yellow/orange 86
full-strength program

acupressure 198, 199,
 200–201, 202–3, 204,
 205
acupuncturist, consulting
 206–7
aromatherapy 209
chakra meditation 212–13
continuing 217–20
copper therapy 214
daily plans 197–216
diet 192–5, 217–19
exercise routine 195–6,
 219
herbalism 211
joint symptoms,
 monitoring 220
reiki 217
shopping list 193
supplements 195, 219

gardening 102
garlic 84, 93
gentle program
 acupressure 129
 aromatherapy 119, 120,
  121, 122, 124, 125, 126
 continuing 136–9
 daily plans 118–36
 diet 113–15, 137–8
 exercise routine 116–17,
  139
 fluid, drinking 115
 hand reflexology 127
 herbalism 131–2
 homeopathy 130
 joint symptoms,
  monitoring 139
 meditation 133
 shopping list 114
 supplements 116, 138–9
 therapies 117, 139
ginger 168
glucosamine 92
gout 17
grapefruit 84, 120
grapes
 chicken, lime and grape
  salad 143
green tea compote 180

A note about the ORAC test:

The ORAC test measures how well the antioxidants in fruit and vegetables can block the breakdown of a chemical (fluorescein) after it's mixed with a strongly oxidant substance (peroxyl radical). Fluorescein is used because it's luminescent, and the intensity of light it emits decreases as it breaks down. This makes it easy to measure how much fluorescein remains intact at set intervals after being in contact with the oxidant and the fruit or vegetable extract. If the food has a low ORAC value, it provides little protection, fluorescein quickly breaks down and the mixture's luminosity decreases. If the food has a high ORAC value, it protects the fluorescein from degradation and the sample remains luminescent for much longer. After measuring the intensity of fluorescence in the mixture every 35 minutes after adding the oxidant, scientists compare the results with those obtained when using different concentrations of a standard antioxidant (trolox). Results are given in units known as "trolox equivalents" or TE.

Author's acknowledgments

I would like to thank my husband, Richard, who willingly provided invaluable back-up and support during those long hours of research and writing. I would also like to thank everyone who has helped in bringing this book to fruition, including Grace Cheetham at Watkins, Judy Barratt and Kesta Desmond – who ensured consistency throughout – and, of course, my inimitable agent, Mandy Little.